ADVANCES IN STEM CELL RESEARCH SERIES

STEM CELL RESEARCH AND SCIENCE: BACKGROUND AND ISSUES

BRENDAN E. AYLESWORTH
EDITOR

Nova Science Publishers, Inc.
New York

For permission to use material from this book please contact us:
Telephone 631-231-7269; Fax 631-231-8175
Web Site: http://www.novapublishers.com

NOTICE TO THE READER

The Publisher has taken reasonable care in the preparation of this book, but makes no expressed or implied warranty of any kind and assumes no responsibility for any errors or omissions. No liability is assumed for incidental or consequential damages in connection with or arising out of information contained in this book. The Publisher shall not be liable for any special, consequential, or exemplary damages resulting, in whole or in part, from the readers' use of, or reliance upon, this material. Any parts of this book based on government reports are so indicated and copyright is claimed for those parts to the extent applicable to compilations of such works.

10065256885
Independent verification should be sought for any data, advice or recommendations contained in this book. In addition, no responsibility is assumed by the publisher for any injury and/or damage to persons or property arising from any methods, products, instructions, ideas or otherwise contained in this publication.

This publication is designed to provide accurate and authoritative information with regard to the subject matter covered herein. It is sold with the clear understanding that the Publisher is not engaged in rendering legal or any other professional services. If legal or any other expert assistance is required, the services of a competent person should be sought. FROM A DECLARATION OF PARTICIPANTS JOINTLY ADOPTED BY A COMMITTEE OF THE AMERICAN BAR ASSOCIATION AND A COMMITTEE OF PUBLISHERS.

Library of Congress Cataloging-in-Publication Data

Stem cell research and science background and issues / editor, Brendan E. Aylesworth.
    p. cm.
Includes index.
"This book consists of public domain documents which have been located, gathered, combined, reformatted, and enhanced with a subject index, selectively edited and bound to provide easy access."
ISBN 978-1-60876-083-1 (softcover)
1. Stem cells--Research--Government policy--United States. I. Aylesworth, Brendan E.
QH588.S83S73955 2009
616'.02774--dc22
                            2009039027

Published by Nova Science Publishers, Inc. ✝ *New York*

Contents

Preface

Human embryonic stem cells are often described as "master cells," able to develop into any other type of cell in the human body. Research on embryonic stem cells has given rise to ethical debates, as the removal of an embryonic stem cell from an embryo typically involves the destruction of that embryo. In 2007, researchers in Japan and the United States published reports that they had successfully induced adult human somatic cells to exhibit characteristics similar to embryonic stem cells. Some have argued that these new induced pluripotent stem cells render embryonic stem cell research unnecessary, while others contend that continued embryonic stem cell research is still important.

Chapter 1- Human embryonic stem cells are often described as "master cells," able to develop into any other type of cell in the human body. Research on embryonic stem cells has given rise to ethical debates, as the removal of an embryonic stem cell from an embryo typically involves the destruction of that embryo. In 2007, researchers in Japan and the United States published reports that they had successfully induced adult human somatic cells to exhibit characteristics similar to embryonic stem cells. Some have argued that these new induced pluripotent stem cells render embryonic stem cell research unnecessary, while others contend that continued embryonic stem cell research is still important.

Restrictions on the federal funding of research using stem cell lines were recently lifted by an executive order issued by President Obama. Pursuant to that order, the National Institutes of Health is directed to issue guidance on human stem cell research within 120 days. This change reversed an existing executive branch policy that limited federal funds to stem cell lines that were already in existence on August 9, 2001, and were derived with the informed consent of the donors; from excess embryos created solely for reproductive purposes; and without any financial inducements to the donors.

In contrast, the federal funding of most methods of human embryonic stem cell procurement is still prohibited by federal legislation. No federal funds may be used for the derivation of stem cell lines from newly destroyed embryos; the creation of any human embryos for research purposes; or cloning of human embryos for any purposes. Recipients of federal funds may also be prohibited from discriminating against individuals who are opposed to stem cell research.

Several bills have been introduced in the 111th Congress that would direct the Secretary of Health and Human Services to conduct and support stem cell research. Some of these bills would appear to sanction continued federal funding of human embryonic stem cell research, while others would not.

Chapter 2 - The central question before Congress in the debate over human stem cell research is how to treat human embryonic stem cell research (ESR), which may lead to lifesaving treatments, but which requires the destruction of embryos. Current federal law and policy address this question primarily through restrictions on federal funding for ESR. The Dickey amendment prohibits the use of Department of Health Human Services (HHS) funds for the creation of human embryos for research purposes or research in which a human embryo or embryos are destroyed, discarded, or knowingly subjected to certain risks of injury or death. The Dickey amendment thus prohibits the use of HHS funds to establish ES lines (line establishment involves embryo destruction), but not to conduct research using established lines. President Obama established current federal ESR policy with a March 9, 2009, executive order: *Removing Barriers to Responsible Scientific Research Involving Human Stem Cells* (Obama policy). The Obama policy authorizes HHS's National Institutes of Health (NIH) to support and conduct responsible, scientifically worthy human stem cell research, including ESR, to the extent permitted by law. It also requires NIH to issue a guidance consistent with the order. The Obama policy reversed one established by President George W. Bush, which had been the first to allow federal ESR funding, but only for a limited number of ES lines.

Congress has several sets of policy options, each one prompting a set of ethical dilemmas. The first set of options involves permitting or expanding federal ESR funding, as proposed in H.R. 872, H.R. 873, and S. 487. One such option is to take no action, allowing the Obama policy to persist. This option would permit federal funding for ESR with a range of lines, and would allow the executive branch to change the ESR policy in the future. Another such option is to enact a law permitting ESR. Even if consistent with the Obama policy, this course would limit the opportunity for the executive branch to change the policy in the future. A final such option involves expanding ESR by eliminating the Dickey amendment, thus allowing the use of federal funds for the establishment of ES lines, and/or for the creation of embryos for ESR. Some supporters this set of options assert that unused frozen embryos that are created for in vitro fertilization (IVF) could be used for federally regulated research instead of being destroyed. Other supporters seek federally regulated and funded research on embryos created specifically for research purposes, which might help to facilitate more targeted research. Critics seek to protect embryos and/or egg donors, and assert that federal funds should not be used for such purposes.

Congress's second set of options involves funding additional research that may eventually generate embryonic stem cells without destroying embryos, as proposed in H.R. 877. Supporters assert that this facilitates research without ethical dilemmas. Critics characterize it as unnecessary, costly, and a diversion from developing treatments. Congress's third set of options involves discouraging ESR via tax measures, or limiting or eliminating it by restricting research funding, banning certain cloning techniques, or giving embryos the Constitutional right to life. Examples include H.R. 110, H.R. 227, H.R. 881, H.R. 1050, H.R. 1654, S. 99, and S. 346. Supporters claim their approaches respect human dignity; critics claim they harm people already living.

Chapter 3 - Embryonic stem cells have the ability to develop into virtually any cell in the body, and may have the potential to treat injuries as well as illnesses, such as diabetes and Parkinson's disease. In January 2009, the Food and Drug Administration approved a request from Geron, a California biotechnology company, to begin a clinical trial involving safety tests of embryonic stem cells in patients with recent spinal cord injuries.

Currently, most human embryonic stem cell lines used in research are derived from embryos produced via in vitro fertilization (IVF). Because the process of removing these cells destroys the embryo, some individuals believe the derivation of stem cells from human embryos is ethically unacceptable. In November 2007, research groups in Japan and the United States announced the development of embryonic stem cell-like cells, called induced pluripotent stem (iPS) cells, via the introduction of four genes into human skin cells. Those concerned about the ethical implications of deriving stem cells from human embryos argue that researchers should use iPS cells or adult stem cells (from bone marrow or umbilical cord blood). However, many scientists believe research should focus on all types of stem cells.

On March 9, 2009, President Barack Obama signed an executive order that reversed the nearly eight-year old Bush Administration restriction on federal funding for human embryonic stem cell research. In August 2001, President

George W. Bush had announced that for the first time, federal funds would be used to support research on human embryonic stem cells, but funding would be limited to "existing stem cell lines." NIH established a registry of 78 human embryonic stem cell lines eligible for use in federally funded research, but only 21 cell lines were available due to technical reasons and other limitations. Over time scientists became increasingly concerned about the quality and longevity of these 21 stem cell lines. These scientists believe that research advancement requires access to new human embryonic stem cell lines.

H.R. 873 (DeGette), the Stem Cell Research Enhancement Act of 2009, was introduced on February 4, 2009. The text of H.R. 873 is identical to legislation introduced in the 110th Congress, H.R. 3 (DeGette), and the 109th Congress, H.R. 810 (Castle). The bill would allow federal support of research that utilizes human embryonic stem cells regardless of the date on which the stem cells were derived from a human embryo. Stem cell lines must meet ethical guidelines established by the NIH, which would be issued within 60 days of enactment. H.R. 872 (DeGette), the Stem Cell Research Improvement Act of 2009, was also introduced on February 4, 2009. It is similar to H.R. 873 in that it adds the same Section 498D, "Human Embryonic Stem Cell Research," to the PHS Act, but it also adds another Section 498E, "Guidelines on Research Involving Human Stem Cells," which would require the Director of NIH to issue guidelines on research involving human embryonic stem cell within 90 days of enactment; updates of the guidelines would be required every three years. S. 487 (Harkin), introduced on February 26, 2009, is the same as H.R. 873, except it has an additional section supporting research on alternative human pluripotent stem cells. It is identical to a bill introduced in the 110th Congress, S. 5 (Reid).

During the 110th Congress, the Senate passed legislation (S. 5) in April 2007 that would have allowed federal support of research that utilizes human embryonic stem cells regardless of the date on which the stem cells were derived from a human embryo. The bill would have also provided support for research on alternatives, such as iPS cells. The House passed the bill in June 2007, and President Bush vetoed it on June 20, 2007. (The 109th Congress passed a similar bill, which also was vetoed by President Bush, the first veto of his presidency; an attempt to override the veto in the House failed.) On the related issue of human cloning, in June 2007 the House failed to pass a bill (H.R. 2560) that would have imposed penalties on anyone who cloned a human embryo and implanted it in a uterus.

Chapter 4 – This is a testimony of Joseph R. Bertino, presented to the House Committee on Energy and Commerce's Subcommittee on Health.

Chapter 5 – This is a testimony of George Q. Daley, presented to House Committee on Energy and Commerce, Subcommittee on Health "Stem cell science: the foundation for future cures."

Chapter 6 – This is a testimony of John K. Fraser, Principal Scientist, Cytori Therapeutics Inc.

Chapter 7 – This is a testimony of John Gearhart, Institute for Cell Engineering, Johns Hopkins Medicine, given before the United States House of Representatives Subcommittee on Health of the Committee on Energy and Commerce.

Chapter 8 – This is a written testimony of Weyman Johnson, Individual living with Multiple Sclerosis, Chairman of the Board, National Multiple Sclerosis Society to Energy and Commerce Committee Subcommittee on Health, United States House of Representatives.

Chapter 9 – This is a testimony of Amit N Patel, Director of Cardiovascular Cell Therapies, before the Subcommittee on Health of the Committee on Energy and Commerce.

Chapter 10 – This is a statement of Douglas T. Rice, Adult Stem Cell Recipient for the heart.

Chapter 11 – This is a testimony of Elias A. Zerhouni, Director, National Institutes of Health, before the Subcommittee on Health Committee on Energy and Commerce, United States House of Representatives.

In: Stem Cell Research and Science   ISBN: 978-1-60876-083-1
Editor: Brenden E. Aylesworth   © 2010 Nova Science Publishers, Inc.

Chapter 1

Legal Issues Related to Human Embryonic Stem Cell Research

Edward C. Liu

Summary

Human embryonic stem cells are often described as "master cells," able to develop into any other type of cell in the human body. Research on embryonic stem cells has given rise to ethical debates, as the removal of an embryonic stem cell from an embryo typically involves the destruction of that embryo. In 2007, researchers in Japan and the United States published reports that they had successfully induced adult human somatic cells to exhibit characteristics similar to embryonic stem cells. Some have argued that these new induced pluripotent stem cells render embryonic stem cell research unnecessary, while others contend that continued embryonic stem cell research is still important.

Restrictions on the federal funding of research using stem cell lines were recently lifted by an executive order issued by President Obama. Pursuant to that order, the National Institutes of Health is directed to issue guidance on human stem cell research within 120 days. This change reversed an existing executive branch policy that limited federal funds to stem cell lines that were already in existence on August 9, 2001, and were derived (1) with the informed consent of the donors; (2) from excess embryos created solely for reproductive purposes; and (3) without any financial inducements to the donors.

In contrast, the federal funding of most methods of human embryonic stem cell procurement is still prohibited by federal legislation. No federal funds may be used for the derivation of stem cell lines from newly destroyed embryos; the creation of any human embryos for research purposes; or cloning of human embryos for any purposes. Recipients of federal funds may also be prohibited from discriminating against individuals who are opposed to stem cell research.

Several bills have been introduced in the 111th Congress that would direct the Secretary of Health and Human Services to conduct and support stem cell research. Some of these bills would appear to sanction continued federal funding of human embryonic stem cell research, while others would not.

Background Information on Human Embryonic Stem Cells

Human embryonic stem cells are often described as "master cells," able to develop into any other type of cell in the human body.[1] Potential sources for human embryonic stem cells include embryos created via *in vitro* fertilization for either research or reproduction; five to nine week old embryos or fetuses obtained through elective abortion; and embryos created through cloning or somatic cell nuclear transfer. Stem cells which are derived from adult tissues, such as umbilical cord blood or bone marrow, are distinct from embryonic stem cells and do not naturally exhibit the same developmental characteristics or behaviors.

In 1998, researchers at the University of Wisconsin isolated cells from a human embryo early in the developmental cycle and developed the first human embryonic stem cell lines.[2] Controversy surrounds the removal of stem cells from human embryos and fetuses because most techniques require the destruction of the embryo during the removal process. However, human embryonic stem cells are regarded as possibly having more therapeutic or research potential than stem cells derived from adult tissue. Whereas embryonic stem cells are often classified as either totipotent[3] or pluripotent,[4] stem cells found in adult sources may only have the capacity to differentiate into a few types of cells.[5]

Recent discoveries may lessen the demand for embryonic stem cells. In 2007, researchers in Japan and the United States published reports that they had successfully induced human somatic cells to exhibit pluripotent characteristics.[6] This advancement notwithstanding, many stem cell researchers continue to argue that embryonic stem cell procurement is necessary in order to provide, among other things, the "gold standard" against which other means of pluripotent stem cell procurement are measured.[7]

Research utilizing human embryonic stem cell lines has focused on the potential that these cells can offer to advance the treatment or mitigation of diseases and conditions and to generate replacement tissues for disfunctioning cells or organs.[8] Examples of research efforts include spinal cord injury, multiple sclerosis, Parkinson's disease, Alzheimer's disease, and diabetes. Researchers also hope to use specialized cells to replace dysfunctional cells in the brain, spinal cord, pancreas, and other organs.[9] In January of 2009, the Food and Drug Administration approved a clinical trial to evaluate a therapy for spinal cord injuries that was developed using embryonic stem cell lines.[10]

Federal Funding of Embryonic Stem Cell Research

Historically, there have been two sequential phases of research involving human embryonic stem cells: (1) research in which stem cells are produced from human embryonic tissue; and (2) research in which embryonic stem cells are used to study human development or illness. As the state of scientific knowledge and expertise has advanced, the federal government has taken various positions regarding the propriety of federally funding research at each stage. Currently, the use of federal funds for embryonic stem cell procurement is prohibited. In contrast, the guidelines governing the use of federal funds to support research using embryonic stem cell lines already in existence are currently being drafted by the National Institutes of Health (NIH).

Restrictions on Federal Funding of Research Using Embryos

While federal law has regulated federal funding of fetal research since 1974,[11] federal funding of embryonic research has only been restricted since 1994, when President Clinton, through an executive directive, prohibited federal funding of such research.[12] Subsequently, in 1996, Congress enacted a legislative ban in the funding measure of the NIH and has continued to pass a similar ban annually since that time.[13]

The congressional ban, often referred to as the Dickey Amendment,[14] prohibits federally appropriated funds from being used for either the creation of human embryos for research purposes or for research in which a human embryo or embryos are destroyed, discarded, or knowingly subjected to risk of injury or death.[15] The ban defined "human embryo or embryos" to include any organism, not protected as a human subject under 45 C.F.R. § 46 (Human Subject Protection regulations) that is derived by fertilization, parthenogenesis, cloning, or any other means from one or more human gametes.[16] As the collection of embryonic stem cells often entails the destruction of or harm to an embryo, the Dickey Amendment effectively forecloses federal funding of embryonic stem cell procurement.[17]

Despite the absence of federal funding, embryonic research has continued with other sources of funding. In 1998, after the inclusion of the Dickey Amendment, landmark developments were recognized by· scientists· at the University of Wisconsin when researchers were able to isolate stem cells from human embryos and coax them to grow into specialized cells.[18] This development led some to question whether federal funds could be used in subsequent research involving these cell lines.

Research on Embryonic Stem Cell Lines under the Dickey Amendment

In January of 1999, the General Counsel of Health and Human Services (HHS) concluded that the Dickey Amendment's prohibitions against the use of HHS appropriated funds for human embryo research would not apply to research using stem cells "because such cells are not a human embryo within the statutory definition."[19] HHS concluded that NIH could fund research that uses stem cells derived from the embryo by private funds. However, because of the language in the Dickey Amendment, NIH could not fund research that derived the stem cells from embryos.

Some Members of Congress strongly opposed HHS's interpretation and believed that the legislative ban covered and prohibited funding such research. In response to this opposition, HHS Secretary Shalala stated in a letter that the definition of embryo used in the HHS legal opinion relied on the definition of embryo in the statute and that the ban applied only to research in which human embryos are discarded or destroyed, but not to research preceding or following "on such projects."[20] Secretary Shalala also noted that "there is nothing in the legislative history to suggest that the provision was intended to prohibit funding for research in which embryos—organisms—are not involved."[21]

NIH published draft guidelines for funding of stem cell research in the Federal Register in December of 1999 and final guidelines were issued in August of 2000.[22] Based upon HHS's interpretation, the guidelines stated that funds could not be used to extract or derive stem cells from an embryo, thereby destroying it. However, studies utilizing pluripotent stem cell lines derived from human embryos could be conducted using NIH funds provided that the cells were derived (1) without federal funds, (2) from human embryos that were created for the purposes of fertility treatment, and (3) were in excess of the clinical need of the individuals seeking such treatment. NIH initiated the applications process, but that process was overtaken by events and a new administration's policy was set forth.

Recent Executive Branch Policies

When President George W. Bush took office in January of 2001, he announced his intent to conduct a review of the stem cell research issue and ordered HHS to review the NIH guidelines issued by the previous administration. During this transition period, NIH suspended its review of applications from researchers seeking federal funds to perform embryonic stem cell research. Subsequently, on August 9, 2001, President Bush announced that federal funds would be available to human embryonic stem cell research on a restricted basis. The new policy would provide federal funds to be used for research only on existing stem cell lines that were already in existence as of the date of the announcement.[23] In identifying the stem cell lines as being eligible for federal funding, President Bush said these embryos, from which the existing stem cell lines were created, had been destroyed previously and could not develop as human beings.

Under the policy announced on August 9, 2001, federal agencies, primarily NIH, would be permitted to fund embryonic stem cell research if certain eligibility criteria were met. Federal funds could only be used for research on existing stem cell lines that were derived (1) with the informed consent of the donors, (2) from excess embryos created solely for reproductive purposes, and (3) without any financial inducements to the donors.[24]

On March 9, 2009, President Obama issued an executive order revoking the restrictions on human embryonic stem cell funding established under the Bush administration. President Obama's executive order also directed the Director of NIH to

> review existing NIH guidance and other widely recognized guidelines on human stem cell research, including provisions establishing appropriate safeguards, and issue new NIH guidance on such research that is consistent with this order.[25]

Such guidelines must be issued within 120 days of the date of the executive order.

Recent Congressional Activity

Congressional interest in stem cell research continued steadily since President Bush's policy announcement in 2001. Despite the introduction of various bills to both promote and limit federal funding of stem cell research, there exists no legislative enactment defining what types of postprocurement embryonic stem cell research are eligible to receive federal funding.

During the 109th Congress, at least seven bills involving stem cell research were introduced, two of which were enacted.[26] A third measure, H.R. 810, the Stem Cell Research Enhancement Act of 2005, was passed by Congress, but vetoed by President Bush on July 19, 2006.[27] H.R. 810 would have amended the Public Health Service Act (PHSA) to direct the Secretary of HHS to conduct and support research that utilizes human embryonic stem cells without regard to the date on which the stem cells were derived from a human embryo. To be eligible for use in research conducted or supported by the Secretary, the stem cells would have been required to meet certain conditions. For example, only stem cells derived from human embryos that were donated from in vitro fertilization clinics, were created for the purposes of fertility treatment, and were in excess of the clinical need of the individuals seeking such treatment would have been eligible for use.[28] A vote to override the veto was unsuccessful.[29]

Finally, S. 2754, the Alternative Pluripotent Stem Cell Therapies Enhancement Act, would have amended the PHSA to direct the Secretary of HHS to conduct and support basic and applied research to develop techniques for the isolation, derivation, production, or testing of stem cells that are not derived from a human embryo. S. 2754 indicated that the research contemplated by the measure would not have affected any policy, guideline, or regulation regarding embryonic stem cell research or human cloning by somatic cell nuclear transfer. S. 2754 was passed by the Senate on July 18, 2006 by a vote 100-0. The House did not vote on the measure.

In the 110th Congress, at least 10 bills involving stem cell research were introduced.[30] H.R. 3, the Stem Cell Research Enhancement Act of 2007, a measure that was identical in language to the Stem Cell Research Enhancement Act of 2005, was passed by the House on January 11, 2007, by a vote of 253-174. A companion measure, S. 5, was passed by the Senate on April 11, 2007, by a vote of 63-34. S. 5 included the language of H.R. 3, as well as the language of the Alternative Pluripotent Stem Cell Therapies Enhancement Act from the 109th Congress. On June 7, 2007, the House passed S. 5 by a vote of 247-176, but it was ultimately vetoed by President Bush.[31]

In the 111th Congress, H.R. 872, the Stem Cell Research Improvement Act of 2009, contains language that is largely similar to the earlier Stem Cell Research Enhancement Acts of 2005 and 2007, and would amend the PHSA to direct the Secretary of HHS to conduct and support research involving embryonic stem cell lines that met the same criteria enumerated in the prior bills. This bill would additionally require guidelines governing such research to be issued by the Director of NIH within 90 days of enactment, and periodically reviewed every three years. H.R. 873, the Stem Cell Research Enhancement Act of 2009, would also amend the PHSA to direct the Secretary of HHS to conduct and support the same type of embryonic stem cell research. This bill would also require guidelines to be issued within 60 days of enactment, but would not require further periodic review of those guidelines. S. 487, also entitled the Stem Cell Research Enhancement Act of 2009, is identical to S. 5 in the 110th Congress.

Other bills introduced during the 111th Congress are aimed at supporting some types of stem cell research, but appear to exclude most embryonic stem cell research. H.R. 877, the Patients First Act of 2009 would direct the Secretary of HHS to conduct and support research on pluripotent stem cells, but appears to exclude research upon stem cell lines that were derived from embryonic sources. S. 99, the Ethical Stem Cell Research Tax Credit Act of 2009, would provide businesses a credit equal to 30% of "qualified stem cell research expenses."[32] Qualified stem cell research expenses do not appear to include embryonic stem cell procurement activities, insofar as those activities would subject a human embryo to destruction, discarding, or risk of injury. Research activities using embryonic stem cell lines that were derived in a manner which subject a human embryo to destruction, discarding, or risk of injury would not appear to be eligible for the tax credit proposed by this bill.

Conscience Protections

Federal law protects individuals from being required to perform or assist in the performance of federally funded research that is morally or religiously objectionable to them.[33] This protection, which would likely encompass objections to research on embryonic stem cell lines, is only triggered in instances where the objectionable research is federally funded.[34] Therefore it is unlikely to arise in the context of embryonic stem cell procurement, as federal funds may not be used for those purposes.

Facilities that receive biomedical or behavioral research grants are additionally prohibited from discriminating among any employment or staff privileges based upon an individual's opinions of, or prior refusals to participate in, health services or research activities that are contrary to his religious beliefs or moral convictions.[35] This would appear to prevent recipients of NIH grants from discriminating against individuals that are opposed to stem cell research.

In December of 2008, the Bush administration issued final regulations reiterating these protections and additionally requiring recipients of federal funds to certify, in writing, that they will refrain from these prohibited actions.[36] The Obama administration has indicated that it intends to rescind these regulations.[37]

End Notes

[1] In contrast, differentiated somatic cells, which perform the "day to day" functions of the body, are not thought to give rise to other types of cells absent human intervention. *See, e.g., infra* footnote 6 and accompanying text.

[2] Nat'l Inst. of Health, U.S. Dep't of Health & Hum. Services, *Stem Cells: Scientific Progress and Future Research Directions* 4 (2001), *available at* http://stemcells.nih.gov/info/scireport/2001report.htm.

[3] The earliest embryonic stem cells are called totipotent cells as they can develop into an entire organism, producing both the embryo and tissues required to support it in the uterus. PRESIDENT'S COUNCIL ON BIOETHICS, *Alternative Sources of Human Pluripotent Stem Cells*, at 5 n.* (2005), *available at* http://www.bioethics.gov.

[4] Pluripotent stem cells can develop into almost any type of cell in the body, but these stem cells cannot form the supporting tissues necessary for gestation, as seen with totipotent cells. *Id.*

[5] For example, hematopoietic stem cells found in adult bone marrow and umbilical cord blood only appear to naturally give rise to various types of blood cells. PRESIDENT'S COUNCIL ON BIOETHICS, *Monitoring Stem Cell Research*, at 3 (2004), *available at* http://www.bioethics.gov.

[6] James A. Thomson et al., *Induced Pluripotent Stem Cell Lines Derived from Human Somatic Cells*, 318 SCIENCE 1917 (2007); Shinya Yamanaka et al., *Induction of Pluripotent Stem Cells from Adult Human Fibroblasts by Defined Factors*, 131(5) CELL 861 (2007).

[7] Robert Lee Holtz, *Stem-Cell Researchers Claim Embryo Labs Are Still a Necessity*, THE WALL ST. J., Jan. 4, 2008, at B1.

[8] For additional information on stem cell research, see CRS Report RL33540, *Stem Cell Research: Federal Research Funding and Oversight*, by Judith A. Johnson and Erin D. Williams.

[9] *Id.* at 4-6.

[10] Andrew Pollack, *Milestone in Research in Stem Cells*, NEW YORK TIMES, Jan. 23, 2009, at 1.

[11] National Research Service Award Act of 1974, P.L. 93-348, § 213, 88 Stat. 342 (1974).

[12] Statement on Federal Funding of Research on Human Embryos, 30 Weekly Comp. Pres. Doc. 2459 (December 2, 1994).

[13] Balanced Budget Downpayment Act, 1996, P.L. 104-99, § 128, 110 Stat. 26, 34 (1996).

[14] The amendment is so named for its principal sponsor, Rep. Jay Dickey.

[15] This term was defined as risk greater than that allowed for research on fetuses in utero under 45 C.F.R. § 46.208(a)(2) and 42 U.S.C. § 289g(b).

[16] The rider language has not changed significantly over the years and is currently found in Title V of the Labor, HHS, and Education appropriations acts. P.L. 110-161,§ 509 (2007).

[17] *But see* CRS Report RL33554, *Stem Cell Research: Ethical Issues*, by Erin D. Williams and Judith A. Johnson, at 14-15 (discussing potential methods of creating embryonic stem cell lines without destroying human embryos).

[18] James A. Thomson et al., *Embryonic Stem Cell Lines Derived from Human Blastocysts*, 282 SCIENCE 1145 (1998).

[19] Letter from HHS Gen. Counsel Harriet Rabb to Harold Varmus, Director, NIH, January 15, 1999. General Counsel Rabb determined that the statutory ban on human embryonic research defined an embryo as an "organism" that, when implanted in the uterus, is capable of becoming a human being. The opinion stated that pluripotent stem cells are not, and cannot, develop into an organism, as defined in the statute.

[20] Letter from Secretary Shalala to Rep. Jay Dickey, February 23, 1999.

[21] *Id.*

[22] 64 Fed. Reg. 67,576 (Dec. 2, 1999); 65 Fed. Reg. 51,976 (Aug. 25, 2000).

[23] President's Address to the Nation on Stem Cell Research From Crawford, Texas, 37 Weekly Comp. Pres. Doc. 1149 (August 9, 2001).

[24] *Id.* The policy also required the creation of the President's Council on Bioethics to study stem cells and embryonic research as well as other issues.

[25] Exec. Order No. _____, § 3, Mar. 9, 2009, *available at* http://www.whitehouse.gov/the_press_office/Removing-Barriers-to-Responsible-Scientific-Research-Involving-Human-Stem-Cells/.

[26] H.R. 2520, 109th Cong., Stem Cell Therapeutic and Research Act of 2005 (providing for the collection and maintenance of human cord blood stem cells) (enacted as P.L. 109-129). S. 3504, 109th Cong., Fetus Farming Prohibition Act of 2006 (making it unlawful to either solicit or knowingly acquire, receive, or accept a donation of human fetal tissue knowing that a human pregnancy was deliberately initiated to provide such tissue or obtained from a human embryo or fetus that was gestated in the uterus of a nonhuman animal) (enacted as P.L. 109-242).

[27] A companion bill, S. 471, was introduced by Sen. Arlen Specter on February 28, 2005.

[28] The President argued that the bill would compel taxpayers "to fund the deliberate destruction of human embryos," and that "crossing this line would ... needlessly encourage a conflict between science and ethics that can only do damage to both and harm our Nation as a whole." 152 Cong. Rec. H5435 (daily ed. July 19, 2006) (Stem Cell Research Enhancement Act of 2005—Veto Message From the President of the United States (H. Doc. No. 109-127)).

[29] *See* 152 Cong. Rec. H5450 (daily ed. July 19, 2006) (the vote was 235-193).

[30] For additional discussion of stem cell research legislation in the 110th Congress, see CRS Report RL33540, *Stem Cell Research: Federal Research Funding and Oversight*, by Judith A. Johnson and Erin D. Williams, supra footnote 8 at 25-29.

[31] Message to the Senate of the United States (June 20, 2007), *available at* http://www.whitehouse.gov/news/releases/2007/06/print/20070620-5.html. The President observed, "S. 5, like the bill I vetoed last year, would overturn today's carefully balanced policy on stem cell research. Compelling American taxpayers to support the deliberate destruction of human embryos would be a grave mistake."

[32] This bill is similar to S. 2863 in the 110th Congress.

[33] 42 U.S.C. § 300a-7(d).

[34] *Id.*

[35] 42 U.S.C. § 300a-7(c)(2).

[36] 45 C.F.R. §§ 88.4(d), 88.5. *See* 73 Fed. Reg. 78,071-101.

[37] *See* Rob Stein, *Health Workers' Conscience Rule Set to Be Voided*, WASHINGTON POST, Feb. 28, 2009, at A1.

In: Stem Cell Research and Science   ISBN: 978-1-60876-083-1
Editor: Brenden E. Aylesworth   © 2010 Nova Science Publishers, Inc.

Chapter 2

Stem Cell Research: Ethical Issues

Erin D. Williams and Judith A. Johnson

Summary

The central question before Congress in the debate over human stem cell research is how to treat human embryonic stem cell research (ESR), which may lead to lifesaving treatments, but which requires the destruction of embryos. Current federal law and policy address this question primarily through restrictions on federal funding for ESR. The Dickey amendment prohibits the use of Department of Health Human Services (HHS) funds for the creation of human embryos for research purposes or research in which a human embryo or embryos are destroyed, discarded, or knowingly subjected to certain risks of injury or death. The Dickey amendment thus prohibits the use of HHS funds to establish ES lines (line establishment involves embryo destruction), but not to conduct research using established lines. President Obama established current federal ESR policy with a March 9, 2009, executive order: *Removing Barriers to Responsible Scientific Research Involving Human Stem Cells* (Obama policy). The Obama policy authorizes HHS's National Institutes of Health (NIH) to support and conduct responsible, scientifically worthy human stem cell research, including ESR, to the extent permitted by law. It also requires NIH to issue a guidance consistent with the order. The Obama policy reversed one established by

President George W. Bush, which had been the first to allow federal ESR funding, but only for a limited number of ES lines.

Congress has several sets of policy options, each one prompting a set of ethical dilemmas. The first set of options involves permitting or expanding federal ESR funding, as proposed in H.R. 872, H.R. 873, and S. 487. One such option is to take no action, allowing the Obama policy to persist. This option would permit federal funding for ESR with a range of lines, and would allow the executive branch to change the ESR policy in the future. Another such option is to enact a law permitting ESR. Even if consistent with the Obama policy, this course would limit the opportunity for the executive branch to change the policy in the future. A final such option involves expanding ESR by eliminating the Dickey amendment, thus allowing the use of federal funds for the establishment of ES lines, and/or for the creation of embryos for ESR. Some supporters this set of options assert that unused frozen embryos that are created for in vitro fertilization (IVF) could be used for federally regulated research instead of being destroyed. Other supporters seek federally regulated and funded research on embryos created specifically for research purposes, which might help to facilitate more targeted research. Critics seek to protect embryos and/or egg donors, and assert that federal funds should not be used for such purposes.

Congress's second set of options involves funding additional research that may eventually generate embryonic stem cells without destroying embryos, as proposed in H.R. 877. Supporters assert that this facilitates research without ethical dilemmas. Critics characterize it as unnecessary, costly, and a diversion from developing treatments. Congress's third set of options involves discouraging ESR via tax measures, or limiting or eliminating it by restricting research funding, banning certain cloning techniques, or giving embryos the Constitutional right to life. Examples include H.R. 110, H.R. 227, H.R. 881, H.R. 1050, H.R. 1654, S. 99, and S. 346. Supporters claim their approaches respect human dignity; critics claim they harm people already living.

It details the ethical arguments that surround ESR. The broadest is the balance of embryo destruction and relief of human suffering. More subtle issues focus on the relative importance of the viability of embryos, the purpose of embryo creation, new versus existing cell lines, the consent of donors, the ethics of egg procurement, the effectiveness of alternatives, the possibility of generating embryonic stem cells without destroying human embryos, and the use of federal funding.

Introduction

Human stem cell research is controversial not because of its goals, but rather because of the means of obtaining some of the cells. Research involving most types of human stem cells, such as those derived from adult tissues and umbilical cord blood, has been uncontroversial, except when its effectiveness as an alternative to embryonic stem cells is debated. The crux of the debate centers around embryonic stem cells, which enable research that may facilitate the development of medical treatments and cures, but which require the destruction of an embryo to derive.[1] In addition, because cloning is one method of producing embryos for research, the ethical issues surrounding cloning are also relevant.

Current Policy

Federal regulation of human embryonic stem cell research (ESR) primarily consists of one law and one policy: the Dickey amendment and the Obama policy, respectively.[2] Both address the use of federal funding to support ESR. Neither restricts or regulates ESR conducted solely with private, local and/or state government funding, or with funding from other non-federal sources. The Dickey Amendment, the Obama policy, and also the previous policy, which had been established by the George W. Bush Administration, are discussed below.

The Dickey Amendment

Since FY1996, the Dickey amendment, a provision added to each year's Labor-Health and Human Services-Education appropriations legislation, has prohibited the use of Department of Health and Human Services (HHS) funds for the creation of human embryos for research purposes or research in which a human embryo or embryos are destroyed, discarded, or knowingly subjected to risk of injury or death greater than that allowed for research on fetuses in utero under 45 CFR 46.204(b). This policy effectively precludes the use of federal funding to derive stem cells from embryos, which typically are produced via in vitro fertilization (IVF). However, the extracted embryonic stem cells can be used to generate embryonic stem cell lines that may continue to divide for many months to years. According to a legal opinion issued by the HHS General Council in 1999, by contrast to funding restrictions that Dickey places on the derivation of stem cells from embryos, federal funding for research performed with embryonic stem cells themselves (which does not itself involve embryos or the extraction of

stem cells from embryos) is not proscribed by the Dickey amendment.[3] It is
funding for research with these embryonic stem cell lines that is the subject of the
Obama policy and of much of the current legislation before Congress.

The Obama Policy

The Obama policy took effect on March 9, 2009, in the form of an executive
order.[4] In the executive order, President Barack Obama authorized the HHS
Secretary, including the National Institutes of Health (NIH), to support and
conduct responsible, scientifically worthy human stem cell research, including
human embryonic stem cell research, to the extent permitted by law. The
executive order also directed the NIH to review existing NIH guidance and other
widely recognized guidelines on human stem cell research, including provisions
establishing appropriate safeguards, and issue new NIH guidance on such
research that is consistent with the executive order within 120 days (by early July
2009). On the same day that the executive order was issued, President Obama
issued a memorandum on scientific integrity directing the head of the White
House Office of Science and Technology Policy "to develop a strategy for
restoring scientific integrity to government decision making."[5]

Historical Note: The Bush Policy

Prior to the Obama policy, ESR had been regulated by the policy that
President George W. Bush had established in August 2001 (Bush policy). The
Bush policy had, for the first time, allowed federal money to be used to support
ESR. It had also restricted that funding to research using ES lines created (1) with
appropriate informed consent of the donors, (2) using embryos created for
reproductive purposes, and (3) before the date of the policy. This date restriction
was the most controversial component of the Bush policy. President Bush had
later issued a companion policy in the form of *Executive Order: Expanding
Approved Stem Cell Lines in Ethically Responsible Ways* (E.O. 13435), which
had directed the NIH to fund research on sources of pluripotent stem cells that did
not involve the destruction of embryos.[6] President Bush had issued E.O. 13435 on
June 20, 2007, which was the same day that he vetoed a bill to expand federal
funding for ESR (S. 5, 110th).

The Obama policy reversed the Bush policy, and also revoked E.O. 13435.
The Obama policy thus allowed for the possibility of federal funding for ESR
using many more stem cell lines than were previously eligible. While the Obama
policy did not mandate funding for alternatives to ESR, it specifically authorized
support for non-embryonic as well as embryonic stem cell research.

Legislation

Since ESR emerged bringing hope for medical cures and fears about ethical implications, a number of bills have been introduced that touch upon the subject. Enactment of any of these bills, even if consistent with the current executive policy, would limit or eliminate the opportunity for the executive branch to set the ESR policy in the future.

One set of bills would enact into law the authority to expend federal funds on ESR. Some of these bills were introduced prior to the Obama policy, and include restrictions greater than of those Obama policy. For example, some bills require that embryos used in federally funded ESR have been created for reproductive purposes, and/or that there have been no financial inducements made to embryo donors. However, none of these bills contains the August 2001 date restriction that had been imposed by the Bush policy. Examples of these bills in the 111th Congress include H.R. 872, H.R. 873, and S. 487.

A second set of bills would create incentives for activities that avoid ESR. Some of these bills would require federal support or tax benefits for research or activities that avoid damaging embryos. Others would create additional oversight for the conduct of ESR. Still others would create a bank of non-embryonic stem cells from amniotic fluid and placentas. Examples of these bills in the 111th Congress include H.R. 877, S. 99, and H.R. 1654.

A third set of bills would further restrict or prohibit ESR. Some would accomplish this through legislation placing the language of the Dickey amendment in statute, and/or extending it by prohibiting federal funding using stem cells derived in violation of the other restrictions. Others would allow funding only in very specific circumstances, such as when using techniques with non-living embryos created for reproductive purposes. Still others would amend other law (such as that governing the right to life, organ transplantation,[7] cloning, or the creation of animal-human hybrids) to prohibit ESR or restrict some aspect its conduct. Examples of such bills in the 111th Congress include H.R. 110, H.R. 227, H.R. 881, H.R. 1050, and S. 346.

Along with the policy options articulated in the above bills, Congress has additional options thathave been discussed in various forums. One of these is eliminating the Dickey amendment, thus allowing the use of federal funds for the establishment of ES lines, and/or for the creation of embryos for ESR. Another is to take no action, thus allowing the Obama policy to persist. This option would permit federal funding for ESR with a range of lines, and would allow the executive branch some latitude to change the ESR policy in the future.

Proponents and Opponents

In the ES debate, the Obama Administration, George W. Bush Administration (Bush Administration), a group of Representatives, a group of Senators, and a group of Nobel Laureates have each presented their respective positions on ESR. In addition, various other organizations, individuals, and councils have issued opinions and reports on the topic. Some groups, such as the National Academies,[8] the Coalition for the Advancement of Medical Research (CAMR),[9] former First Lady Nancy Reagan,[10] former Presidents Gerald Ford, Jimmy Carter, and Bill Clinton,[11] and the Union of Orthodox Jewish Congregations of America (UOJCA),[12] favor federal support ESR that is generally keeping with the Obama policy. Other groups, such as the Christian Legal Society,[13] Focus on the Family,[14] and the Christian Coalition[15] favor restrictions on ESR, and had supported the Bush policy. Still others, such as the National Right to Life Committee[16] and the United States Conference of Catholic Bishops,[17] oppose all ESR.

Two presidential bioethics advisory panels have considered the issues involved in ESR. The President's Council on Bioethics (President's Council)[18] published one report directly on the topic, *Monitoring Stem Cell Research*,[19] in which it sought to characterize the issues. While the Council made no recommendations there, in two other reports it has recommended that "Congress should ... [p]rohibit the use of human embryos in research beyond a designated stage in their development (between 10 and 14 days after fertilization),"[20] and unanimously recommended "a ban on cloning-to-produce-children," with a 10-member majority also favoring "a four-year moratorium on cloning-for-biomedical-research," and a seven-member minority favoring "regulation of the use of cloned embryos for biomedical research."[21] More recently, the President's Council published Alternative Sources of Human Pluripotent Stem Cells, a white paper exploring the ethics of four proposals to attempt to generate human embryonic stem cells "without creating, destroying, or harming human embryos."[22] A predecessor to the President's Council, the National Bioethics Advisory Commission (NBAC),[23] recommended federal funding for stem cell research using "embryos remaining after infertility treatments," but not for the "derivation or use of embryos ... made for research purposes."[24]

Discussion of Ethical Issues

Detailed review of the assorted reports and statements reveals that while positions on ESR may be broadly categorized as *for* or *against*, there is an array of finer distinctions present. These finer distinctions, in turn, reveal the variation in ethical and moral as well as factual beliefs. The following discussion breaks down the arguments about ESR according to these finer distinctions, demonstrating both the complexity of the issues and the points of resonance among the groups.

Embryo Destruction and Relief of Human Suffering

Most positions on ESR rest at least in part on the relative moral weight accorded to embryos and that accorded to the prospect of saving, prolonging, or improving others' lives. For some, the inquiry begins and ends with this question. For instance, one opponent of the research, the American Life League, posits that "human life begins at conception/fertilization and that there is never an acceptable reason for intentionally taking an innocent human life."[25] Similarly, the United States Conference of Catholic Bishops states that the research is immoral because it "relies on the destruction of some defenseless human beings for the possible benefit to others."[26]

Some groups explore the moral standing of human embryos, and also consider the "duty to relieve the pain and suffering of others."[27] Others take the position that embryos do not have the same moral status as persons. They acknowledge that embryos are genetically human, but hold that they do not have the same moral relevance because they lack specific capacities, including consciousness, reasoning, and sentience.[28] They also argue that viewing embryos as persons would "rule out all fertility treatments that involve the creation and discarding of excess embryos," and further assert that we do not have the same "moral or religious" response to the natural loss of embryos (through miscarriage) that we do to the death of infants.[29] Some have also rooted their arguments in religious texts, which inform them that an "isolated fertilized egg does not enjoy the full status of person-hood and its attendant protections."[30] They conclude that performing research to benefit persons justifies the destruction of embryos. Acceptance of the notion that the destruction of embryos can be justified in some circumstances forms the basis of pro-ESR opinions—including those of the Bush and Obama Administrations—and is usually modified with some combination of the distinctions and limitations that follow.

Viability of Embryos

Some proponents of ESR base their support on the question of whether an embryo is viable. The relevance of the viability distinction rests on the premise that it is morally preferable for embryos that will not grow or develop beyond a certain stage and/or those that would otherwise be discarded to be used for the purpose of alleviating human suffering.

The Obama policy does not reference the viability of embryos, but allows for the possibility that NIH guidance will do so. By contrast, the Bush policy had directly referenced viability, requiring, among other things, use of stem cells derived from only excess (non-viable) embryos for federally funded research. One report of the President's Council explores the moral significance of viability that is based upon "human choices" rather than an embryo's "own intrinsic nature," but draws no conclusions.[31] A second report broaches the subject of viability, recommending that Congress ban both the transfer of a human embryo to a woman's uterus for any purpose other than to produce a live-born child, and also research conducted on embryos more than 10 to 14 days after fertilization.[32] The NBAC report touches on the moral status of embryos in utero and those in vitro,[33] though NBAC does not specify whether viability was a key rationale for its recommendations. A group of Representatives,[34] a group of Senators,[35] and CAMR imply but do not state a distinction based on viability by expressly calling for the use of "excess" embryos developed for IVF, and making no mention of those in utero.[36] UOJCA makes a similar argument in its letter. By contrast, the National Academies and the group of Nobel Laureates more broadly support research on embryos, making no mention of viability.

Purpose of Embryo Creation

A separate distinction that often leads to the same conclusions as viability is the purpose for which embryos are created. This distinction draws an ethical line based upon the intent of the people creating embryos. In the view of some, it is permissible to create an embryo for reproductive purposes (such as IVF), but impermissible to create one with the intention of destroying it for research. Others worry that moral lines will erode quickly—from using only "spare" embryos left over in fertility clinics to creating human embryos solely for research to creating (or trying to create) cloned embryos solely for research.[37]

As is the case regarding embryo viability, the Obama policy does not reference the purpose of embryo creation, but allows for the possibility that NIH guidance will do so. Most groups at least note the potential ethical significance of reproductive versus research motives for creating embryos. The Bush policy had drawn a motive distinction by including a requirement that federally funded research be conducted only on embryonic stem cell lines derived from embryos created solely for reproductive purposes. NBAC draws the same distinction by recommending that federal funding be used for embryos remaining after infertility treatment but not for research involving the derivation or use of stem cells from embryos made for research purposes or from cloned embryos produced by SCNT.[38] UOJCA argue similarly that they "believe it is entirely appropriate to utilize for this research existing embryos, such as those created for IVF purposes that would otherwise be discarded but for this research. We think it another matter to create embryos ab initio for the sole purpose of conducting this form of research."[39]

The President's Council recommends that Congress ban attempts at conception by any means other than the union of egg and sperm (essentially banning cloning via SCNT) but does not specify whether embryos might be created in vitro specifically for research purposes.[40] Two Council members expressed a dissenting opinion in a medical journal article, arguing that SCNT "resembles a tissue culture" and that the products of SCNT should be available for research.[41] A group of Representatives, a group of Senators, and CAMR imply but do not state that embryos should not be created for research purposes. They overtly call for the use of "excess" embryos developed for IVF and make no mention of embryos created expressly for research.[42] By contrast, the National Academies supports the creation of embryos for research purposes, including via cloning (SCNT), to "ensure that stem cell-based therapies can be broadly applied for many conditions and people [by] overcoming the problem of tissue rejection."[43] Mrs. Nancy Reagan, her supporters, and the group of Nobel Laureates also take this position.

New and Existing Cell Lines

A further distinction has been drawn based upon the timing of the creation of embryonic stem cell lines. Here, the premise is that it is unacceptable to induce the destruction of embryos for the creation of new lines. However, in cases in which embryos have already been destroyed and the lines already exist, it is morally preferable to use those lines for research to improve the human condition.

The Obama policy makes no distinction based on the timing of when ES lines were created. By contrast, the timing of ES-line creation was one central concept in the Bush policy, which had limited the use of federal funding to research on lines derived on or before the date of the policy. Supporters of a distinction based on timing favor this distinction as a compromise because allows research on some embryonic stem cell lines and deters the future destruction of embryos for research. The President's Council writes that a policy based on timing mixes "prudence" with "principle, in the hope that the two might reinforce (rather than undermine) each other."[44] The Council notes that a timing-based policy is supported by what it titled a *moralist's* notion of when one may benefit from prior bad acts (referring to embryo destruction): it prevents the government from complying in the commission of or encouraging the act in the future, and it reaffirms the principle that the act was wrong.[45] The same report also contains alternative analyses that characterize the act of drawing a distinction between new and existing cell lines as "arbitrary," "unsustainable," and "inconsistent."[46] The Council itself takes no position in the report on this or any other issue.

Opponents of any distinction based on timing come from both sides of the issue. They view the distinction between new and existing stem cell lines with reproach. One side, which includes the National Right to Life Committee and the United States Conference of Catholic Bishops, objects because the distinction validates destruction of embryos, and rewards those who did so first with a monopoly. The other side, which includes the National Academies, a group of Representatives, a group of Senators, Nancy Reagan and her supporters, Gerald Ford, CAMR, and the group of Nobel Laureates, objects because the distinction limits the number of embryonic stem cell lines available for research, particularly since the number of authorized lines are dwindling[47] and are "contaminated with mouse feeder cells."[48] Likewise, though NBAC recognized the distinction between destroying embryos and using ones previously destroyed (e.g., "derivation of [embryonic stem] cells involves destroying the embryos, whereas abortion precedes the donation of fetal tissue and death precedes the donation of whole organs for transplantation"),[49] it still recommended future development of embryonic stem cell lines. UOJCA also recognizes a distinction between new and existing lines: "research on embryonic stem cells must be conducted under careful guidelines [that] ... relate to where the embryonic stem cells to be researched upon are taken from."[50]

Consent of Donors

There is consensus throughout a wide array of viewpoints about ESR that embryos should only be obtained for research with the consent of their biological donors. This consent requirement necessitates that embryos be taken only with donors' knowledge, understanding, and uncoerced agreement, which may, in fact, be complicated by conflicting studies regarding the long-term health effects of egg donation.[51] The donor consent requirement is consistent with the rules governing human beings' participation in research, and with individuals' general legal authority to make decisions regarding embryos they procreate. A potential drawback of the requirement is that it may restrict the number of embryos available for research purposes.

While the Obama policy does not explicitly require the consent of the donors, it does require that NIH support ESR conducted responsibly, which may include informed consent requirements.[52] The Bush policy had contained a donor consent requirement that had limited approved stem cell lines to those derived with the informed consent of the donors, and obtained without any financial inducements to the donors. Despite the policy, a 2008 report raised questions about whether one quarter of the lines eligible for federal funding actually met policy's the informed consent requirements.[53]

Like the Bush policy, the NBAC, the President's Council, and the UOJCA also favor donor consent requirements. The National Academies notes the importance of informed consent in its discussion of stem cell research oversight requirements.[54] A group of Representatives and a group of Senators mention and imply their support for donor consent requirements.[55]

Egg Procurement

Egg procurement from women has raised a number of issues, most notably, those of informed consent and payment. The topic of informed consent in egg procurement came to the public's attention in November 2005 with allegations that some human eggs used in South Korean scientist Dr. Hwang's laboratory had been obtained under coercive conditions. Informed consent can be undermined when a coercive situation prevents a free choice from being made, or when insufficient information is provided to the person making a decision. The situation alleged in Dr. Hwang's laboratory raises the issue of coercion both because subordinate women in the laboratory allegedly donated eggs, and because some women were allegedly paid for their eggs. A 2002 study conducted by a University of Pennsylvania student raised the issue of insufficient information, finding that a number of programs seeking donor eggs for reproductive purposes downplayed the risks involved in egg retrieval.[56] The wide consensus regarding the need for informed consent necessarily implies similar consensus on the need for an information-rich, coercion-free method of obtaining eggs, however there is some disagreement on the specifics of whether payment for eggs necessarily constitutes coercion.

Paying women for their eggs, which has been debated in the context of seeking donor eggs both for reproductive purposes (for example, to enable women who do not produce their own eggs to become pregnant), and for research purposes, is not unheard of in the United States. According to a 2000 study by the American Society of Reproductive Medicine (ASRM), some IVF programs reportedly offered as much as $5,000 for one egg retrieval cycle, though $2,500 appeared to be a more common amount.[57] Offers of much higher amounts ($50,000-$100,000) have been reported elsewhere.[58] Dr. Huang's laboratory reportedly made payments of $1,400 to each woman who donated eggs.[59] Payments are not illegal in the Unites States, nor were they illegal in South Korea at the time Dr. Huang's laboratory allegedly made them. The questions are, is payment for egg donation ever acceptable, and if so, what amount is appropriate?

Several arguments have been put forth in favor of payment for egg donation, many focused on donation for reproductive purposes.[60] First, some have argued that payment creates incentives to increase the number of egg donors, thus facilitating research and benefitting infertile couples. Second, some reason that payment for eggs gives women parity with sperm donors, who may be compensated for donating gametes at a lower rate given that they require a much less involved procedure. In addition, some argue that participants should be offered an amount commensurate with the time, inconvenience, discomfort, and risks of the procedure, as is the general practice in biomedical research.[61] Third, some allege that fairness dictates that women who donate eggs ought to be able to benefit from their action. Fourth, some claim that pressures created by financial incentives may be no greater than those experienced by women asked to make altruistic egg donations for relatives or friends, and may thus not rise to the level of coercion. These are the types of arguments that led ASRM to recommend in

2000 that sums of up to $5,000 may be appropriate for typical egg donation, while sums of up to $10,000 may possibly be justified if there are particular difficulties a woman must endure to make her donation.

Several arguments have also been put forth against payment for egg donation. First, some voiced fears that payment might lead to the exploitation of women, particularly poor women, and the commodification of reproductive tissues.[62] Second, some have argued that payment for eggs for research purposes might undermine public confidence in endeavors such as human ESR.[63] Arguments such as these have prompted both the National Academies and the President's Council to recommend that women not be paid for donating their eggs for research purposes. It also led the President's Council to note that in theory, there is the possibility that eggs could be procured from ovaries harvested from cadavers, which might at least alleviate concerns related to coercion.

It is worth noting that a woman may choose to undergo egg retrieval for her own reproductive purposes, which would effectively take the process of egg procurement out of the research arena and avoids the question of payment entirely. (For example, this could be an option for a woman seeking IVF because her fallopian tubes are blocked). While not making specific recommendations about payment for research-related egg donation, several groups' recommendations that only embryos left over from IVF procedures be used for stem cell research (noted above in the *Purpose of Embryo Creation* section) effectively takes the process of egg procurement from women out of the research arena. As is the case regarding other issues, the Obama policy does not reference the topic of egg donation, but allows for the possibility that NIH guidance will do so. The Bush policy had kept the consent process for egg retrieval separate from donation by funding research only on lines derived from embryos originally created for fertility treatments.

Effectiveness of Alternatives

One factual distinction that has been used to support competing ethical viewpoints is the efficacy of alternatives to ESR. The promise of stem cell therapies derived from adult tissue and umbilical cord blood have buttressed opposition to ESR. A report that stem cells similar to embryonic stem cells can be found in amniotic fluid may do the same, although the lead scientist conducting research on the amniotic cells and others have stated that amniotic cells will not make embryonic stem cells irrelevant.[64] Perhaps more promising, scientists claim to have generated pluripotent stem cells from adult cells, though technical and safety concerns regarding the cells' therapeutic use remain unresolved.[65] Alternatives such as those proposed for consideration by the President's Council are discussed in the next section. Some opponents of the current method of obtaining embryonic stem cells argue that therapies and cures can be developed without the morally undesirable destruction of embryos. The Obama policy neither requires not precludes research into ESR alternatives on its face, but does require that research be responsible and scientifically worthy. By contrast, E.O. 6/20 had affirmatively directed the pursuit of alternative methods of deriving embryonic stem cells, implying both a belief in the promise and necessity of such actions.

Not all scientists agree that adult stem cells or pluripotent stem cells derived from adult tissue hold as much potential as embryonic stem cells. Notably, during a congressional subcommittee hearing, when the NIH Director, Dr.. Elias Zerhouni, was asked if other avenues of research should be pursued instead, he stated that "the presentations about adult stem cells holding as much or more potential than embryonic stem cells, in my view, do not hold scientific water. I think they are overstated."[66] Concerns have been raised that pluripotent stem cells derived from adult tissue may not be as versatile as embryonic stem cells, and may induce tumors.[67] Most supporters of ESR believe that it is the quickest and, perhaps in some cases, the only path that will yield results. Supporters also stress that embryonic and other stem cell research should be conducted collaboratively, so that they can inform one another. On a related note, some have pointed out that benefits from one alternative to ESR, umbilical cord blood banking, may only be available to families who can afford to pay private companies' storage fees.

Findings regarding the effectiveness of alternatives to ESR are mixed. The President's Council notes that there is a "debate about the relative merits of embryonic stem cells and adult stem cells."[68] Focus on the Family cites promising non-embryonic stem cell research: "adult stem cells may be as 'flexible' as embryonic ones and equally capable of converting into various cell types for healing the body."[69] By contrast, the National Academies finds that the "best available scientific and medical evidence indicates that research on both embryonic and adult human stem cells will be needed."[70] NBAC finds in its deliberations that "the claim that there are alternatives to using stem cells derived from embryos is not, at the present time, supported scientifically."[71] CAMR supports both embryonic and adult stem cell research, and adds that "many scientists believe and studies show that embryonic stem cells will likely be more effective in curing diseases because they can grow and differentiate into any of the body's cells and tissues and thus into different organs."[72] Mrs. Nancy Reagan and her supporters favor expedient approaches including ESR.[73]

Several laws have supported the development of stem cells from sources other than embryos. For each of fiscal years 2004 through 2006, Congress allocated money in the HHS appropriations for the establishment and continuation of a National Cord Blood Stem Cell Bank within the Health Resources and Services Administration. In 2005, Congress enacted P.L. 109-129 for the collection and maintenance of human cord blood stem cells for the treatment of patients and for research.

Generating Embryonic Stem Cells without Destroying Human Embryos

One possible alternative to ESR as it has typically been conducted, the ability to generate embryonic stem cells without destroying human embryos, was explored by the President's Council in its 2005 white paper,[74] described in the introductory section of this report. The white paper discusses four potential methods of obtaining embryonic stem cells without having to destroy embryos. Those methods, the scientific and practical merits of which remain far from settled, are (1) extracting cells from organismically dead embryos; (2) non-harmful biopsy of living embryos; (3) bioengineering embryo-like artifacts; and (4) dedifferentiating somatic cells.[75]

In the white paper, the President's Council examined the ethical acceptability of each method. The first two seek to avoid the destruction of embryos either by developing standards for declaring an embryo "dead" when its cells have stopped dividing or by removing a cell from an embryo without destroying the embryo itself. The other two methods would avoid having to use an embryo altogether, by attempting to obtain embryonic stem cells through the destruction of something that is not an embryo.

The Council concluded that the use of organismically dead embryos raises a number of ethical questions that have yet to be answered. They include whether it is possible to be certain that an embryo is really dead, whether the proposal would put embryos at additional risk, and whether IVF practitioners would be encouraged to create extra embryos. A September 2006 report that a team based in Serbia and England had derived stem cells from "dead" embryos prompted precisely these types of questions, as well some regarding whether the stem cells might carry some defect that had made the embryos non-viable.[76]

Regarding the use of non-harmful biopsy, the Council found that it would be ethically unacceptable to test in humans because risks should not be imposed on living embryos destined to become children for the sake of getting stem cells for research. This same response was prompted by an August 2006 report in the journal *Nature* that a California company had used the nonharmful biopsy method to derive stem cells.[77] In addition, the technique was criticized on one side for effectively "creating a twin and then killing that twin,"[78] and on the other for being an inefficient method for deriving stem cell lines.[79] In November 2006, *Nature* issued an addendum to the August article to clarify that, while the company's lead scientist maintained that his method could be used to derive stem cells without destroying embryos, in fact, he had destroyed all of the embryos during his own experiments.[80]

The Council also concluded that bioengineering embryo-like artifacts raises many serious ethical concerns, including whether the artifact would really be a very defective embryo, the ethics of egg procurement, concerns about the use of genetic engineering itself, and the possibility of its use creating a "slippery slope." Finally, the Council found the proposal to dedifferentiate somatic cells to be ethically acceptable if and when it became scientifically practical, provided that de facto embryos were not created.

Although some Council members expressed their support for efforts to identify means of obtaining human embryonic stem cells for biomedical research that do not involve killing or harming human embryos, not all of the members agreed. Some expressed concern that all four methods would "use financial resources that would be better devoted to proposals that are likely to be more productive." One member wrote that he did not support publishing the white paper "with the implied endorsement that special efforts be made in the scientific areas described. While some of the suggestions could be explored in a scientific setting, most are high-risk options that only have an outside chance of success and raise their own complex set of ethical questions."

As is generally the case regarding alternatives to ESR, on its face the Obama policy neither requires not precludes funding research to obtain ES without destroying embryos, but does require that research be responsible and scientifically worthy. By contrast, E.O. 6/20 had specifically directed the HHS Secretary to consider the techniques outlined by the President's Council, and to fund attempts to generate sources of pluripotent stem cell therapies that were not derived from human embryos.

Use of Federal Funding

Some division over the support for and opposition to ESR focuses on the question of whether the use of federal funding is appropriate. Those who oppose federal funding argue that the government should not be associated with embryo destruction.[81] They point out that embryo destruction violates the "deeply held moral beliefs of some citizens," and suggest that "funding alternative research is morally preferable."[82] Proponents of federal funding argue that it is immoral to discourage life-saving research by withholding federal funding. They point out that consensus support is not required for many federal spending policies, as it "does not violate democratic principles or infringe on the rights of dissent of those in the minority."[83] They argue that the efforts of both federally supported and privately supported researchers are necessary to keep the United States at the forefront of what they believe is a very important, cutting edge area of science. Furthermore, supporters believe that the oversight that comes with federal dollars will result in better and more ethically controlled research in the field. Requirements attached to federal funding are one traditional mechanism that Congress has used to regulate scientific research that might otherwise be conducted without federal oversight.[84]

Groups' positions on federal funding tend to mirror their positions on stem cell research generally. The Obama policy authorizes federal funding for ESR, and requires funded research be responsible and scientifically worthy. The Bush policy had also authorized federal funding, but not in a way designed to effect how stem cell lines were established.[85] The President's Council does not take a position on the issue, but notes the pros and cons and stresses that there is a "difference between *prohibiting* embryo research and *refraining from funding* it."[86] Focus on the Family opposes ESR, including federal funding for it.[87] NBAC finds the arguments in favor of federal funding more persuasive than those against it.[88] The National Academies, a group of Representatives, a group of Senators, Mrs. Nancy Reagan and her supporters, CAMR, the Nobel Laureates, and the UOJCA favor federal funding for ESR.[89]

End Notes

[1] For an overview of various religious perspectives on embryonic stem cell research, see LeRoy Walters, "Human Embryonic Stem Cell Research: An Intercultural Perspective," *Kennedy Institute of Ethics Journal*, vol. 14, no. 1, March 2004, p. 3.

[2] For further information, see CRS Report RL33540, *Stem Cell Research: Federal Research Funding and Oversight*, by Judith A. Johnson and Erin D. Williams.

[3] For further information about the Dickey amendment and the HHS General Council's opinion, see CRS Report RL33540, *Stem Cell Research: Federal Research Funding and Oversight*, by Judith A. Johnson and Erin D. Williams.

[4] "Removing Barriers to Responsible Scientific Research Involving Human Stem Cells," March 9, 2009, at http://www.whitehouse.gov/the_press_office/Removing-Barriers-to-Responsible-Scientific-Research-Involving-Human-Stem-Cells/.

[5] The White House, Office of the Press Secretary, Remarks of President Barack Obama-As Prepared for Delivery, Signing of Stem Cell Executive Order and Scientific Integrity Presidential Memorandum, March 9, 2009, at http://www.whitehouse.gov/the_press_office/Remarks-of-the-President-As-Prepared-for-Delivery-Signing-of-Stem-Cell-Executive-Order-and-Scientific-Integrity-Presidential-Memorandum/.

[6] George W. Bush, Executive Order: Expanding Approved Stem Cell Lines in Ethically Responsible Ways, June 20, 2007, at http://www.whitehouse.gov/news/releases/2007/06/20070620-6.html.

[7] For further information about 42 U.S.C. 274e and valuable consideration, see CRS Report RL33902, *Living Organ Donation and Valuable Consideration*, by Erin D. Williams, Bernice Reyes-Akinbileje, and Kathleen S. Swendiman.

[8] The National Academies brings together "committees of experts in all areas of scientific and technological endeavor" as "advisors to the Nation." For statements on ESR and cloning, see National Research Council, Institute of Medicine, National Academies, *Stem Cells and the Future of Regenerative Medicine* (Washington: National Academies, 2001); and Committee on Science, Engineering and Public Policy and Global Affairs Division, et al., *Scientific and Medical Aspects of Human Reproductive Cloning* (Washington, National Academy Press, 2002) at http://www.nationalacademies.org/about/#org.

[9] CAMR was formed in 2001 to ensure that the voices of patients, scientists, and physicians were heard in the debate over stem cell research and the future of regenerative medicine http://www.camradvocacy.org/about_us.aspx; visited January 18, 2007. For a statement on ESR, see Coalition for the Advancement of Medical Research, "The Promise of Embryonic Stem Cells, http://www.camradvocacy.org/resources/The_Promise_of_Embryonic_Stem_Cells.htm, visited Jan 18, 2007.

[10] "Nancy Reagan plea on stem cells," *BBC News*, May 10, 2004, at http://news.bbc.co.uk/2/hi/americas/3700015.stm, visited January 18, 2007; Letter from Nancy Reagan to Senator Orrin Hatch, May 1, 2006, at http://www.camradvocacy.org/resources/Nancy_Reagan.pdf, visited January 18, 2007.

[11] Ibid.

[12] Letter from Harvey Blitz, President, UOJCA et al., to President George W. Bush, July 26, 2001, at http://www.ou.org/public/statements/2001/nate34.htm, visited July 14, 2005. (Hereafter cited as UOJCA letter.)

[13] The Christian Legal Society is a "national grassroots network of lawyers and law students, committed to ... advocating biblical conflict reconciliation, public justice, religious freedom and the sanctity of human life." At http://www.clsnet.org/clsPages/vision.php, visited July 15, 2005.

[14] *Focus on the Family* was founded in 1977 by Dr. James Dobson to promote the teachings of Jesus Christ. See http://www.family.org.

[15] The Christian Coalition is "the largest and most active conservative grassroots political organization in America," at http://www.cc.org.

[16] The National Right to Life Committee was founded in 1973 to "restore legal protection to innocent human life," at http://www.nrlc.org/Missionstatement.htm.

[17] The United States Conference of Catholic Bishops "is an assembly of the hierarchy of the United States and the U.S. Virgin Islands who jointly exercise certain pastoral functions on behalf of the Christian faithful of the United States," at http://www.usccb.org/whoweare.shtml.

[18] The *President's Council* was created by President Bush in November 2001 to "advise the President on bioethical issues that may emerge as a consequence of advances in biomedical science and technology." George W. Bush, "Creation of The President's Council on Bioethics," Executive Order 13237, November 28, 2001.

[19] The President's Council on Bioethics, *Monitoring Stem Cell Research*, January 2004.

[20] The President's Council on Bioethics, *Reproduction and Responsibility*, March 2004, p. xlviii.

[21] The President's Council on Bioethics, Human Cloning and Human Dignity, July 2002, pp. xxxv-xxxviii). Note: At the June 20, 2002, meeting, 9 of 17 Council members voted to support cloning for medical research purposes, without a moratorium, provided a regulatory mechanism was established. Because one member of the Council had not attended the meetings and was not voting, the vote seemed to be 9 to 8 in favor of research cloning. However, draft versions of the Council report sent to Council members on June 28, 2002, indicated that 2 of the group of 9 members had changed their votes in favor of a moratorium. Both made it clear that they have no ethical problem with cloning for biomedical research, but felt that a moratorium would provide time for additional discussion. The changed vote took many Council members by surprise, and some on the Council believe that the moratorium option, as opposed to a ban, was thrown in at the last minute and did not receive adequate discussion. In addition, some on the Council believe that the widely reported final vote of 10 to 7 in favor of a moratorium does not accurately reflect the fact "that the majority of the council has no problem with the ethics of biomedical cloning." (Transcripts of the Council meetings and papers developed by staff for discussion during Council meetings can be found at http://www.bioethics.gov; S. S. Hall, "President's Bioethics Council Delivers," *Science*, vol. 297, July 19, 2002, pp. 322-324.) "Wise Words from Across the Pond?," *BioNews*, no. 252, March 29, 2004.

[22] The President's Council on Bioethics, *Alternative Sources of Human Pluripotent Stem Cells* (May 2005), at http://www.bioethics.gov/reports/white_paper/index.html, visited July 14, 2005.

[23] In 1995, President Clinton created the National Bioethics Advisory Commission by Executive Order, to advise him on bioethical issues. The Order expired in 2001. "Former Bioethics Commissions," *President's Commission on Bioethics* website, at http://www.bioethics.gov/reports/past_commissions/index.html, visited June 30, 2004.

[24] National Bioethics Advisory Commission, *Ethical Issues in Human Stem Cell Research*, vol. 1, September 1999, pp. 70-71.

[25] American Life League, *The Bush Stem Cell Decision*, 2001, athttp://www.all.org/article.php?id=10746& search=2001,visited January 18, 2007.

[26] Office of Communications, United States Conference of Catholic Bishops, *Catholic Bishops Criticize Bush Policy on Embryo Research* (August 9, 2001), at http://www.usccb.org/comm/archives/2001/01-142.shtml.

[27] The President's Council on Bioethics, *Monitoring Stem Cell Research*, January 2004, pp. 58, 62.

[28] Presentation by B. Steinbock, Department of Philosophy, SUNY, Albany, NY, NIH Human Embryo Research Panel Meeting, February 3, 1994.

[29] Michael Sandel, "Embryo Ethics—The Moral Logic of Stem-Cell Research," *New England Journal of Medicine*, vol. 351, no. 3, July 15, 2004, p. 208.

[30] UOJCA letter.

[31] The President's Council on Bioethics, *Monitoring Stem Cell Research*, January 2004, p. 87.

[32] The President's Council on Bioethics, *Reproduction and Responsibility*, March 2004.

[33] National Bioethics Advisory Commission, *Ethical Issues in Human Stem Cell Research*, vol. 1, September 1999, p. 50.

[34] Letter from 206 Members of the House of Representatives to President George W. Bush, April 28, 2004, at http://www.house.gov/degette/news/releases/040428.pdf. (Hereafter cited as Letter from 206 Members of the House of Representatives.)

[35] Letter from 58 Senators to President George W. Bush, June 7, 2004, at http://feinstein.senate.gov/04Releases/ rstemcell-ltr.pdf. (Hereafter cited as Letter from 58 Senators.)

[36] International Society for Stem Cell Research, "Alternative Methods of Producing Stem Cells: No Substitute for Embryonic Stem Cell Research," *Press Release*, (August 2, 2005), at http://www.isscr.org/press_releases/camr_alternatives.htm, visited April 10, 2007.

[37] See, e.g., Eric Cohen and Robert George, "Stem Cells Without Moral Corruption: Congress Can Give Research a Boost Without Supporting the Misuse of Human Embryos," *Washington Post*, July 6, 2006, p. A21.

[38] National Bioethics Advisory Commission, *Ethical Issues in Human Stem Cell Research*, vol. 1, September 1999, pp. 70-72. In SCNT the nucleus of an egg is removed and replaced by the nucleus from a mature body cell, such as a skin cell obtained from a patient. In 1996, scientists in Scotland used the SCNT procedure to produce Dolly the sheep, the first mammalian clone.

[39] UOJCA letter.

[40] The President's Council on Bioethics, *Reproduction and Responsibility*, March 2004, p. xlviii.

[41] Paul McHugh, "Zygote and 'Clonote'—The Ethical Use of Embryonic Stem Cells," *New England Journal of Medicine*, vol. 351, no. 3, July 15, 2004, p. 210.

[42] Letter from 206 Members of the House of Representatives; Letter from 58 Senators.

[43] National Research Council, Institute of Medicine, National Academies, *Stem Cells and the Future of Regenerative Medicine* (Washington: National Academies, 2001), p. 58.

[44] The President's Council on Bioethics, *Monitoring Stem Cell Research*, January 2004, pp. 33-34.

[45] Ibid.

[46] The President's Council on Bioethics, *Monitoring Stem Cell Research*, January 2004, pp. 63-67.

[47] Bridget M. Kuehn, "Genetic Flaws Found in Aging Stem Cell Lines," *Journal of the American Medical Association*, vol. 294, no. 15 (October 2005), p. 1883.

[48] Letter from 206 Members of the House of Representatives; Letter from 58 Senators.

[49] National Bioethics Advisory Commission, *Ethical Issues in Human Stem Cell Research*, vol. 1, September 1999, p. 49.

[50] UOJCA letter.

[51] Kathy Hudson, "International Society for Stem Cell Research Draft Guidelines," *Genetics & Public Policy Center ENews,* Issue 10 (July 2006), available online at http://www.dnapolicy. org/news.enews.article.nocategory.php? action=detail&newsletter_id=13&article_id=31.

[52] The HHS regulations that generally require informed consent for research involving human subjects research do not generally apply to gametes, embryos, or other tissue, once donated or discarded. (See 45 C.F.R. § 46, subparts A & B.)

[53] See the "Consent of Donors" section of this report for more information.

[54] National Research Council, Institute of Medicine, National Academies, *Stem Cells and the Future of Regenerative Medicine* (Washington: National Academies, 2001), p. 53.

[55] Letter from 206 Members of the House of Representatives; Letter from 58 Senators.

[56] "Egg Donation Ethics Study Wins Award," *Research at Penn*, (March 7, 2005), at http://www.upenn.edu/researchatpenn/article.php?113&soc, visited December 5, 2005.

[57] American Society of Reproductive Medicine, "Financial Incentives in Recruitment of Oocyte Donors," *Fertility and Sterility*, vol. 74, no. 2 (August 2000), p. 216.

[58] See e.g., "Egg Donation Ethics Study Wins Award," *Research at Penn*, (March 7, 2005), at http://www.upenn.edu/researchatpenn/article.php?113&soc, visited December 5, 2005.

[59] James Brooke, "Korean Leaves Cloning Center in Ethics Furor," Professional Ethics website (November 25, 2005), at http://ethics.tamucc.edu/article.pl?sid=05/11/26/1524206&mode=t hread visited December 12, 2005.

[60] Unless otherwise noted, these arguments can be found, among other places, at American Society of Reproductive Medicine, "Financial incentives in recruitment of oocyte donors," *Fertility and Sterility*, vol. 74, no. 2 (August 2000), p. 218; and Claudia Kalb, "Ethics, Eggs and Embryos," *MSNBC.com, Newsweek website*, at http://www.msnbc.msn.com/id/8185339/site/newsweek/, visited December 12, 2005.

[61] Kathy Hudson, "International Society for Stem Cell Research Draft Guidelines," *Genetics & Public Policy Center ENews*, Issue 10 (July 2006), available online at http://www.dnapolicy. org/news.enews.article. nocategory.php?action=detail&newsletter_id=13&article_id=31.

[62] See e.g., President's Council on Bioethics, *White Paper: Alternative Sources of Pluripotent Stem Cells* (May 2005), pp. 40-41 at http://www.bioethics.gov/reports/white_paper/index.html, visited December 12, 2005.

[63] National Academies, *Guidelines for Human Embryonic Stem Cell Research*, (Washington, DC: National Academies Press, p. 87, at http://books.nap.edu/books/0309096537/html/87.html, visited, December 12, 2005.

[64] Rick Weiss, "Scientists See Potential In Amniotic Stem Cells," *Washington Post*, January 8, 2007, p. A1, at http://www.washingtonpost.com/wp-dyn/content/article/2007/01/07/AR2007010 700674. html, visited January 8, 2007.

[65] Junying Yu et al., "Induced Pluripotent Stem Cell Lines Derived from Human Somatic Cells," *Science*, vol. 318, no. 5858 (21 December 2007; originally published in *Science Express* on 20 November 2007).

[66] Dr. Elias Zerhouni's answer to a question during the "Fiscal 2008 budget for the National Institutes of Health," *Hearing of the U.S. Senate Appropriations Subcommittee on Labor, Health and Human Services, Education, and Related Agencies* (March 19, 2007).

[67] "The News: Scientists for the first time have generated human stem cells from adult cells," *Bioethics Responder from the Hastings Center*, (20 November 2007).

[68] The President's Council on Bioethics, *Monitoring Stem Cell Research*, January 2004, p. 10.

[69] Carrie Gordon Earll, "Talking Points on Stem Cell Research," *Focus on the Family*, September 17, 2003 at http://www.family.org/cforum/fosi/bioethics/faqs/a0027980.cfm.

[70] National Research Council, Institute of Medicine, National Academies, *Stem Cells and the Future of Regenerative Medicine* (Washington: National Academies, 2001), p. 56.

[71] National Bioethics Advisory Commission, *Ethical Issues in Human Stem Cell Research*, vol. 1, September 1999, p. 53.

[72] Coalition for the Advancement of Medical Research, "The Promise of Embryonic Stem Cells," at http://www.camradvocacy.org/resources/The_Promise_of_Embryonic_Stem_Cells.htm, visited January 18, 2007.

[73] Nancy Reagan plea on stem cells," *BBC News*, May 10, 2004, at http://news.bbc.co.uk/2/hi/ americas/3700015.stm, visited January 18, 2007; Letter from Nancy Reagan to Senator Orrin Hatch, May 1, 2006, at http://www.camradvocacy.org/resources/Nancy_Reagan.pdf, visited January 18, 2007.

[74] The President's Council on Bioethics, *White Paper: Alternative Sources of Human Pluripotent Stem Cells*, May 2005, online at http://www.bioethics.gov/reports/white_paper/index.html.

[75] For more information, see CRS Report RL33540, *Stem Cell Research: Federal Research Funding and Oversight*, by Judith A. Johnson and Erin D. Williams.

[76] See, e.g., Rick Weiss "Researchers Report Growing Stem Cells From Dead Embryos," *Washington Post*, September 23, 2006, p. A03, available online at http://www.washingtonpost.com/wp-dyn/content/article/2006/09/22/AR2006092201377.html.

[77] See e.g., Nicholas Wade, "Stem Cell News Could Intensify Political Debate," *New York Times*, August 24, 2006, available online at http://www.nytimes.com/2006/08/24/science/ 24stem.html?ex=1164862800&en =1d51ef92cddc3e82&ei=5070.

[78] Ibid.

[79] See e.g., Josephine Quintavalle, "The Lanza Protocol: Damned With Very Faint Praise," *BioNews*, vol. 373, (August 22-28, 2006), available online at http://www.bionews.org.uk/commentary. lasso?storyid=3157.

[80] Robert Laza et al., "Human Embryonic Stem Cell Lines Derived from Single Blastomeres," *Nature*, vol. 444, p. 481 (November 23, 2006), available online at http://www.nature.com/nature/journal/v444/n7118/ full/nature05366.html.

[81] National Bioethics Advisory Commission, *Ethical Issues in Human Stem Cell Research*, vol. 1, September 1999, p. 57.

[82] Ibid.

[83] Ibid.

[84] For further information about Congressional regulation of research involving human subjects, see CRS Report RL32909, *Federal Protection for Human Research Subjects: An Analysis of the Common Rule and Its Interactions with FDA Regulations and the HIPAA Privacy Rule*, by Erin D. Williams.

[85] Because the Bush policy only allowed funding for work with previously established ES lines, researchers who had created stem cell lines before the policy took effect could not have been influenced by its ethical constraints regarding the derivation of stem cells from embryos, as their work preceded the policy. Similarly, researchers who created stem cell lines after the policy took effect would not have been motivated to follow the Bush policy's ethical guidelines regarding the creation of stem cell lines, because the results of their work would have remained ineligible for federal funding regardless of their methodology. By contrast, E.O. 6/20 may have affected the future derivation of embryonic stem cells to the extent that it encouraged that such activities take place without creating embryos for research or harming, endangering, or destroying them.

[86] The President's Council on Bioethics, *Monitoring Stem Cell Research*, January 2004, p. 37.

[87] *Stem Cell Research: Our Position (Stem Cells)*, Focus on The Family, 2009,http://www.focusonthe family.com/socialissues/sanctity_of_life/stem_cell_research/our_position.aspx. The group had previously expressed general support for President Bush and his ESR policy, but was "disappointed by his decision to allow federal funding of research on the existing stem cell lines." Carrie Gordon Earll, "Talking Points on Stem Cell Research," *Focus on the Family*, September 17, 2003 at http://www.family.org/cforum/fosi/bioethics/faqs/a0027980.cfm.

[88] National Bioethics Advisory Commission, *Ethical Issues in Human Stem Cell Research*, vol. 1, September 1999, p. 70.

[89] See, e.g., National Research Council, Institute of Medicine, National Academies, *Stem Cells and the Future of Regenerative Medicine* (Washington: National Academies, 2001), p. 49.

In: Stem Cell Research and Science
Editor: Brenden E. Aylesworth

ISBN: 978-1-60876-083-1
© 2010 Nova Science Publishers, Inc.

Chapter 3

Stem Cell Research: Federal Research Funding and Oversight

Judith A. Johnson and Erin D. Williams

Summary

Embryonic stem cells have the ability to develop into virtually any cell in the body, and may have the potential to treat injuries as well as illnesses, such as diabetes and Parkinson's disease. In January 2009, the Food and Drug Administration approved a request from Geron, a California biotechnology company, to begin a clinical trial involving safety tests of embryonic stem cells in patients with recent spinal cord injuries.

Currently, most human embryonic stem cell lines used in research are derived from embryos produced via in vitro fertilization (IVF). Because the process of removing these cells destroys the embryo, some individuals believe the derivation of stem cells from human embryos is ethically unacceptable. In November 2007, research groups in Japan and the United States announced the development of embryonic stem cell-like cells, called induced pluripotent stem (iPS) cells, via the introduction of four genes into human skin cells. Those concerned about the ethical implications of deriving stem cells from human embryos argue that researchers should use iPS cells or adult stem cells (from bone marrow or umbilical cord blood). However, many scientists believe research should focus on all types of stem cells.

On March 9, 2009, President Barack Obama signed an executive order that reversed the nearly eight-year old Bush Administration restriction on federal funding for human embryonic stem cell research. In August 2001, President George W. Bush had announced that for the first time, federal funds would be used to support research on human embryonic stem cells, but funding would be limited to "existing stem cell lines." NIH established a registry of 78 human embryonic stem cell lines eligible for use in federally funded research, but only 21 cell lines were available due to technical reasons and other limitations. Over time scientists became increasingly concerned about the quality and longevity of these 21 stem cell lines. These scientists believe that research advancement requires access to new human embryonic stem cell lines.

H.R. 873 (DeGette), the Stem Cell Research Enhancement Act of 2009, was introduced on February 4, 2009. The text of H.R. 873 is identical to legislation introduced in the 110th Congress, H.R. 3 (DeGette), and the 109th Congress, H.R. 810 (Castle). The bill would allow federal support of research that utilizes human embryonic stem cells regardless of the date on which the stem cells were derived from a human embryo. Stem cell lines must meet ethical guidelines established by the NIH, which would be issued within 60 days of enactment. H.R. 872 (DeGette), the Stem Cell Research Improvement Act of 2009, was also introduced on February 4, 2009. It is similar to H.R. 873 in that it adds the same Section 498D, "Human Embryonic Stem Cell Research," to the PHS Act, but it also adds another Section 498E, "Guidelines on Research Involving Human Stem Cells," which would require the Director of NIH to issue guidelines on research involving human embryonic stem cell within 90 days of enactment; updates of the guidelines would be required every three years. S. 487 (Harkin), introduced on February 26, 2009, is the same as H.R. 873, except it has an additional section supporting research on alternative human pluripotent stem cells. It is identical to a bill introduced in the 110th Congress, S. 5 (Reid).

During the 110th Congress, the Senate passed legislation (S. 5) in April 2007 that would have allowed federal support of research that utilizes human embryonic stem cells regardless of the date on which the stem cells were derived from a human embryo. The bill would have also provided support for research on alternatives, such as iPS cells. The House passed the bill in June 2007, and President Bush vetoed it on June 20, 2007. (The 109th Congress passed a similar bill, which also was vetoed by President Bush, the first veto of his presidency; an attempt to override the veto in the House failed.) On the related issue of human cloning, in June 2007 the House failed to pass a bill (H.R. 2560) that would have imposed penalties on anyone who cloned a human embryo and implanted it in a uterus.

Introduction

On March 9, 2009, President Barack Obama signed an executive order reversing the nearly eightyear old Bush Administration restriction on federal funding for human embryonic stem cell research.[1] President George W. Bush had announced on August 9, 2001, that for the first time federal funds would be used to support research on human embryonic stem cells. However, the Bush decision limited funding to research on stem cell lines that had been created prior to the date of the policy announcement.

The Obama executive order directs the National Institutes of Health (NIH) to issue new guidelines for the conduct of human embryonic stem cell research within 120 days of the date of the executive order. The Obama decision will allow scientists to use federal funds for research utilizing the hundreds of human embryonic stem cell lines that have been created since the Bush 2001 policy. NIH anticipates using some of the $10 billion in funds provided by the stimulus package (American Recovery and Reinvestment Act of 2009, P.L. 111-5) for research on human embryonic stem cells under the new guidelines.[2] President Obama also issued a memorandum on scientific integrity directing the head of the White House Office of Science and Technology Policy "to develop a strategy for restoring scientific integrity to government decision making."[3]

In order to codify the Obama stem cell policy and prevent future administrations from reversing it, Members of the 111th Congress have introduced legislation (H.R. 872, H.R. 873, S. 487) and stated their intention to quickly pass a stem cell bill.[4] Similar legislation was twice vetoed by President George W. Bush during the 109th and 110th Congress. However, scientists still will not be able to use federal funds for the derivation of new human embryonic stem cell lines or for research involving somatic cell nuclear transfer (SCNT) using human eggs unless Congress removes the existing Dickey Amendment from appropriations legislation.

Research involving human embryonic stem cells is of concern for some individuals because the stem cells are located inside the embryo, and the process of removing the cells destroys the embryo.[5] Many religious and socially conservative individuals believe the destruction of embryos for the purpose of harvesting embryonic stem cells is morally and ethically unacceptable. They argue that researchers should use other alternatives, such as iPS cells or adult stem cells (both discussed below), instead of embryonic stem cells.

Federal funding for the support human embryonic stem cell research was limited under the Bush 2001 policy. NIH identified 78 human embryonic stem cell lines that would be eligible for use in federally funded research, but most were found to be either unavailable or unsuitable for research. Only 21 cell lines were available under the Bush policy. Over time, scientists became increasingly concerned about the quality and longevity of these 21 stem cell lines. Many believe research advancement requires the use of new human embryonic stem cell lines.

The former Director of NIH, Elias Zerhouni, stated in a hearing on March 19, 2007, before the Senate Labor, Health and Human Services (HHS), Education, and Related Agencies Appropriations Subcommittee that "It's not possible for me to see how we can continue the momentum of science and research with the stem cell lines we have at NIH that can be funded."[6] When asked if other avenues of research should be pursued instead, Dr. Zerhouni stated that "the presentations about adult stem cells holding as much or more potential than embryonic stem cells, in my view, do not hold scientific water. I think they are overstated."[7] He noted that competitors in Europe, China, and India are investing heavily in human embryonic stem cell research. "I think it is important for us not to fight with one hand tied behind our back here. I think it's time to move forward on this area. It's time for policy makers to find common ground, to make sure that NIH does not lose its historical leadership.... To sideline NIH on such an issue of importance in my view is shortsighted."[8] On May 8, 2008, Dr. Zerhouni made similar statements about the need for additional embryonic stem cell lines and the value of pursuing all avenues of stem cells research at a hearing before the House Energy and Commerce Subcommittee on Health.[9]

Several states, such as California, Connecticut, Illinois, Maryland, and New Jersey, responded to the Bush stem cell policy limitations by moving forward with their own initiatives to encourage or provide funding for stem cell research, and many others have considered similar action. Proponents of these state stem cell research initiatives want to remain competitive, as well as prevent the relocation of scientists and biotechnology firms to other states or overseas. However, without the central direction and coordinated research approach that the federal government can provide, many are concerned that the states' actions will result in duplication of research efforts among the states, a possible lack of oversight for ethical concerns, and ultimately a loss of U.S. preeminence in this important area of basic research. States may be reconsidering their funding of stem cell research given the change in federal policy that occurred under the Obama Administration.

The 110th Congress addressed the topic of stem cell research early in the first session. H.R. 3 (DeGette) was introduced on January 5, 2007, with 211 cosponsors, and passed the House on January 11, 2007.[10] The bill would have allowed federal support of research that utilizes human embryonic stem cells regardless of the date on which the stem cells were derived from a human embryo, and thus would have negated the August 2001 Bush stem cell policy limitation. The Senate passed S. 5 (Reid) on April 11, the House passed S. 5 on June 7, and President Bush vetoed the bill on June 20, 2007. S. 5 was the same as H.R. 3 except it has an additional section supporting research on alternative human pluripotent stem cells.[11]

Basic Research and Potential Applications

Most cells within an animal or human being are committed to fulfilling a single function within the body. In contrast, stem cells are a unique and important set of cells that are not specialized. Stem cells retain the ability to become some or all of the more than 200 different cell types in the body, and thereby play a critical role in repairing organs and body tissues throughout life. Although the term stem cells is often used in reference to these repair cells within an adult organism, a more fundamental variety of stem cells is found in the early-stage embryo. Embryonic stem cells may have a greater ability to become different types of body cells than adult stem cells.

Embryonic Stem Cells from IVF Embryos or Fetal Tissue

Embryonic stem cells were first isolated from mouse embryos in 1981 and from primate embryos in 1995. Animal embryos were the only source for research on embryonic stem cells until November 1998, when two groups of U.S. scientists announced the successful isolation of human embryonic stem cells. One group, at the University of Wisconsin, derived stem cells from fiveday-old embryos produced via *in vitro* fertilization (IVF).[12] The work is controversial because the stem cells are located within the embryo and the process of removing them destroys the embryo. Many individuals who are opposed to abortion are also opposed to research involving embryos. The second group, at Johns Hopkins University, derived stem cells with very similar properties from five- to nine-week-old embryos or from fetuses obtained through elective abortion.[13] Both groups reported the human embryos or fetuses were donated for research following a process of informing one or more parents and obtaining their consent. The cells removed from embryos or fetuses were manipulated in the laboratory to create embryonic stem cell lines that may continue to divide for many months to years. The vast majority of research on human embryonic stem cells, both in the United States and overseas, utilizes cell lines derived via the University of Wisconsin method.

Induced Pluripotent Stem (iPS) Cells

In November 2007, two research groups, one at Kyoto University in Japan and the second at the University of Wisconsin, Madison, announced the development of embryonic stem cell-like cells, called induced pluripotent stem (iPS) cells, through the introduction of four genes into human skin cells.[14] Until this breakthrough, the characteristics displayed by the iPS cells were thought to occur only in cells found within the embryo. The research teams accomplished the reprogramming of the adult skin cells by using a retrovirus to transport the four genes into the skin cells. The teams each used a different set of four genes; the Kyoto group has subsequently achieved reprogramming using three genes.[15] The work on human iPS cells is based on earlier studies by the Kyoto group in mouse embryos that identified the genes active in early embryos and then used combinations of these genes to try and reprogram adult mouse cells. The successful mouse reprogramming study, using four mouse genes, was announced in June 2006. The analogous four human genes were used by the Kyoto group on the human skin cells.

Although development of iPS cells may one day lessen the need to study stem cells derived from the human embryo, scientists insist that work on human embryonic stem cells must continue for several reasons.[16] For example, it is unclear whether iPS cells share all the characteristics of embryonic stem cells, and therefore multiple comparisons between the two types of cells will be necessary. In addition, because scientists have used potentially cancer-causing retroviruses to transfer the reprogramming genes, these iPS cells would not desirable for therapeutic uses in patients. Therefore, alternative mechanisms to accomplish reprogramming would need to be developed. Scientists are in the process of investigating the use of other safer viruses to transfer the genes. Some groups are exploring chemical methods of achieving the same results by switching on genes in the adult cell rather than transferring in additional gene copies with a virus.

Embryonic Stem Cells Obtained via SCNT (Cloning)

Another potential source of embryonic stem cells is somatic cell nuclear transfer (SCNT), also referred to as cloning.[17] For certain applications, stem cells derived using SCNT may offer the best hope for understanding and treating disease. In SCNT the nucleus of an egg is removed and replaced by the nucleus from a mature body cell, such as a skin cell obtained from a patient. In 1996, scientists in Scotland used the SCNT procedure to produce Dolly the sheep, the first mammalian clone.[18] When SCNT is used to create another individual, such as Dolly, the process is called reproductive cloning. In contrast, scientists interested in using SCNT to create cloned stem cells would allow the cell created via SCNT to develop for a few days, and then the stem cells would be removed for research. Stem cells created via SCNT would be genetically identical to the patient, and thus would avoid any tissue rejection problems that could occur if the cells were transplanted into the patient. Creating stem cells using SCNT for research purposes is sometimes referred to as therapeutic cloning.

Although various scientific groups have reported success in using SCNT to create cloned embryos (which are then used to produce stem cell lines or live births) of a variety of different mammals (sheep, rabbits, cows), attempts at creating primate embryos via SCNT had been unsuccessful. However, in June 2007, researchers at the Oregon National Primate Research Center at Oregon Health and Science University announced the successful derivation of stem cells from a rhesus monkey embryo created via SCNT.[19] Results of the Oregon group were confirmed in November 2007.[20]

The unsubstantiated announcement by Clonaid in December 2002 of the birth of a cloned child have contributed to the controversy over research on human embryos.[21] More recently, charges of ethical and scientific misconduct have clouded the reputation of scientists involved in deriving stem cells from human embryos created via SCNT. In February 2004, scientists at the Seoul National University (SNU) in South Korea announced the first isolation of stem cells from a cloned human embryo and in May 2005 announced advances in the efficiency of creating cloned human embryos and in isolating human stem cells. Concerns about the SNU work arose in November 2005 when a U.S. co-author of the 2005 paper accused Hwang Woo Suk, the lead SNU researcher, of ethical misconduct.[22] In December 2005, a Korean co-author of the May 2005 paper stated that the research was fabricated and the paper should be retracted; Hwang agreed to the retraction. On January 10, 2006, SNU stated that results of the 2004 paper were also a deliberate fabrication.[23] Despite these difficulties, scientists in a number of labs are continuing to work on deriving patient-matched stem cells from cloned human embryos.[24]

Stem Cells from Adult Tissue or Umbilical Cord Blood

Stem cells obtained from adult organisms are also the focus of research. In April 2007, researchers in Brazil published a preliminary report on attempts to treat 15 newly diagnosed type 1 diabetes patients with high-dose immunosuppressive chemotherapy followed by transplantation of the patient's own stem cells.[25] Although this experiment was first proposed by U.S. scientists, the risks associated with the procedure were judged to be to high (5% mortality) for a treatable disease that affects children.[26] Type 1 diabetes is thought to be an autoimmune disease in which the patient's immune system attacks the insulin-producing cells in the pancreas. Scientists are not certain about the exact mechanism of how the treatment works. One hypothesis is that the chemotherapy suppresses the patient's immune system and stops the destruction of the remaining insulin-producing cells in the patient's body, which is why early diagnosis is crucial in this approach. The patient's stem cells are then transfused back into the body, hopefully becoming part of an immune system that will not continue to attack the patient's insulin-producing cells.

A January 2007 report found that cells similar to embryonic stem cells can be found in amniotic fluid. However, the lead author of the report, as well as others in the field, caution that these cells are not a replacement for embryonic stem cells.[27] There have been a number of other publications on the abilities and characteristics of adult stem cells from a variety of different sources, such as bone marrow and the umbilical cord following birth. Bone marrow transplantation, a type of adult stem cell therapy, has been used for 50 years to treat patients for a variety of blood-related conditions.[28] Several private companies (such as MorphoGen, NeuralStem, Osiris Therapeutics, StemSource, ViaCell) are working on additional therapeutic uses of adult stem cells.

In 1999, David A. Prentice of the Family Research Council and other biomedical researchers founded Do No Harm: The Coalition of Americans for Research Ethics, a group that opposes stem cell research on the grounds that it is unethical because it destroys embryos and is unnecessary due to the success of adult stem cell therapy. Do No Harm has compiled a list of 73 diseases that it claims can be treated using adult stem cells.[29] In a July 2006 letter to *Science,* Smith et al. accuse Prentice of misleading the public and deceiving patients with the list because only nine of the adult stem cell treatments have been "fully tested in all required phases of clinical trials and approved by the U.S. Food and Drug Administration."[30] Prentice responded in a January 2007 letter that "Our list of [then] 72 applications, compiled from peer-reviewed articles, documents observable and measurable benefit to patients, a necessary step toward formal FDA approval and what is expected of new, cutting-edge medical applications."[31] Prentice also accused Smith et al. of "cruelly deceiving patients and the public" by promoting the "falsehood that embryonic stem cell cures are imminent." In a June 2007 exchange, Smith et al. continue to emphasize that the majority of treatments on the list haven't met FDA standards.[32] Prentice defended the list by pointing to tangible benefits to some patients.[33] Both sides again accused the other of misleading laypeople and deceiving patients.

Opponents of stem cell research advocate that adult instead of embryonic stem cell research should be pursued because they believe the derivation of stem cells from either IVF embryos or aborted fetuses is ethically unacceptable. Others believe that adult stem cells should not be the sole target of research because of important scientific and technical limitations. Adult stem cells may not be as long lived or capable of as many cell divisions as embryonic stem cells. Also, adult stem cells may not be as versatile in developing into various types of tissue as embryonic stem cells, and the location and rarity of the cells in the body might rule out safe and easy access. For these reasons, many scientists argue that both adult and embryonic stem cells should be the subject of research, allowing for a comparison of their various capabilities. Reports issued by the NIH and the Institute of Medicine (IoM) state that both embryonic and adult stem cell research should be pursued.[34]

In FY2004, the Consolidated Appropriations Act, 2004 (P.L. 108-199) provided $10 million to establish a National Cord Blood Stem Cell Bank within the Health Resources and Services Administration (HRSA). HRSA was directed to use $1 million to contract with the IoM to conduct a study that would recommend an optimal structure for the program. The study, *Cord Blood: Establishing a National Hematopoietic Stem Cell Bank Program,* was released in

April 2005. The blood cell forming stem cells found in cord blood can be used as an alternative to bone marrow transplantation in the treatment of leukemia, lymphoma, certain types of anemia, and inherited disorders of immunity and metabolism. The IOM report provides the logistical process for establishing a national cord blood banking system, establishes uniform standards for cord blood collection and storage, and provides recommendations on ethical and legal issues associated with cord blood collection, storage and use.

On December 20, 2005, the President signed the Stem Cell Therapeutic and Research Act of 2005 (P.L. 109-129). The act provides for the collection and maintenance of human cord blood stem cells for the treatment of patients and for research. It stipulates that amounts appropriated in FY2004 or FY2005 for this purpose shall remain available until the end of FY2007, and authorizes $60 million over FY2007-FY2010. The act also reauthorizes the national bone marrow registry with $186 million over FY2006-FY2010. In addition, it creates a database to enable health care workers to search for cord blood and bone marrow matches and links all these functions under a new name, the C.W. Bill Young Cell Transplantation program.

Potential Applications of Stem Cell Research

Stem cells provide the opportunity to study the growth and differentiation of individual cells into tissues. Understanding these processes could provide insights into the causes of birth defects, genetic abnormalities, and other disease states. If normal development were better understood, it might be possible to prevent or correct some of these conditions. Stem cells could be used to produce large amounts of one cell type to test new drugs for effectiveness and chemicals for toxicity. The damaging side effects of medical treatments might be repaired with stem cell treatment. For example, cancer chemotherapy destroys immune cells in patients, decreasing their ability to fight off a broad range of diseases; correcting this adverse effect would be a major advance. Stem cells might be transplanted into the body to treat disease (e.g., diabetes, Parkinson's disease) or injury (e.g., spinal cord).

In January 2009, the Food and Drug Administration approved a request from Geron, a California biotechnology company, to begin a Phase I clinical trial involving safety tests of embryonic stem cells in 8 to 10 patients with recent spinal cord injuries.[35] In this first human subject trial using embryonic stem cells, the injected cells are intended to "help repair the insulation, known as myelin, around nerve cells, restoring the ability of some nerve cells to carry signals. There is also hope that growth factors produced by the injected cells will spur damaged nerve cells to regenerate."[36] Some scientists have expressed concern over the possibility that the transplanted cells may form a type of tumor called a teratoma, but extensive studies in rodents were performed to assure FDA that the stem cells did not causes tumors in animals.[37]

Before stem cells can be applied to human medical problems, substantial advances in basic cell biology and clinical technique are required. In addition, very challenging regulatory decisions will be required on any individually created tissue-based therapies resulting from stem cell research. Such decisions would likely be made by the Center for Biologics Evaluation and Research (CBER) of the Food and Drug Administration (FDA). The potential benefits mentioned above would be likely only after many more years of research. Technical hurdles include developing the ability to control the differentiation of stem cells into a desired cell type (like a heart or nerve cell) and to ensure that uncontrolled development, such as cancer, does not occur. Some experiments may involve the creation of a chimera, an organism that contains two or more genetically distinct cell types, from the same species or different species.[38] If stem cells are to be used for transplantation, the problem of immune rejection must also be overcome. Some scientists think that the creation of many more embryonic stem cell lines will eventually account for all the various immunological types needed for use in tissue transplantation therapy. Others envision the eventual development of a "universal donor" type of stem cell tissue, analogous to a universal blood donor.

However, if the method used to create iPS cells or if the SCNT technique was employed (using a cell nucleus from the patient), the stem cells created via these methods would be genetically identical to the patient, would presumably be recognized by the patient's immune system, and thus might avoid any tissue rejection problems that could occur in other stem cell therapeutic approaches. Because of this, scientists believe that these techniques may provide the best hope of eventually treating patients using stem cells for tissue transplantation.

Regulation of Research

A Brief History of Federal Policy on Human Embryo Research

Federal funding of *any* type of research involving human embryos, starting with *in vitro* fertilization (IVF) then later the creation of stem cell lines from embryos, had been blocked by various policy decisions dating back 30 years.

Ethics Advisory Board

Following the birth of the first IVF baby, Louise Brown, in July 1978, the federal Ethics Advisory Board (EAB) was tasked with considering the scientific, ethical, legal, and social issues surrounding human IVF.[39] The EAB released its report on May 4, 1979, which found that IVF research was acceptable from an ethical standpoint and could be supported with federal funds. The EAB's recommendations were never adopted by HHS, the EAB was dissolved in 1980, and no other EAB was ever chartered. Because federal regulations that govern human subject research (45 C.F.R. Part 46) stipulated that, at the time, federally supported research involving human IVF must be reviewed by an EAB, a so-called "de facto moratorium" on human IVF research resulted. Other types of embryo research ensuing from the development and use of IVF, such as cloning and stem cells, were therefore also blocked. The de facto moratorium was lifted with the enactment of the National Institutes of Health (NIH) Revitalization Act of 1993 (P.L. 103-43, Section 121(c)), which nullified the regulatory provision (45 C.F.R. § 46.204(d)) requiring EAB review of IVF proposals.

NIH Human Embryo Research Panel

In response, the NIH established the Human Embryo Research Panel to assess the moral and ethical issues raised by this research and to develop recommendations for NIH review and conduct of human embryo research. The NIH Panel released a report providing guidelines and recommendations on human embryo research in September 1994. The panel identified areas of human embryo research it considered to be unacceptable, or to warrant additional review. It determined that certain types of cloning[40] without transfer to the uterus warranted additional review before the panel could recommend whether the research should be federally funded. However, the panel concluded that federal funding for such cloning techniques followed by transfer to the uterus should be unacceptable into the foreseeable future. The NIH Panel recommended that some areas of human embryo research should be considered for federal funding, including SCNT, stem cells and, under certain limited conditions, *embryos created solely for the purpose of research.*[41] The panel's report was unanimously accepted by the NIH Advisory Committee to the Director (ACD) on December 2, 1994.

After the ACD meeting on December 2, 1994, President Clinton directed NIH *not* to allocate resources to support the *"creation of human embryos for research purposes."* The President's directive did not apply to research involving so-called "spare" embryos, those that sometimes remain from clinical IVF procedures performed to assist infertile couples to become parents. Nor did it apply to human parthenotes, eggs that begin development through artificial activation, not through fertilization. Following the Clinton December 2, 1994, directive to NIH, the agency proceeded with plans to develop guidelines to support research using spare embryos. NIH plans to develop guidelines on embryo research were halted on January 26, 1996, with the enactment of P.L. 104-99, which contained a rider that affected FY1996 funding for NIH. The rider, often referred to as the Dickey Amendment, prohibited HHS from using appropriated funds for the creation of human embryos for research purposes or for research in which human embryos are destroyed.

The Dickey Amendment

Prior to an August 2001 Bush Administration decision (see below), no federal funds had been used to support research on stem cells derived from either human embryos or fetal tissue.[42] The work at the University of Wisconsin and Johns Hopkins University was supported by private funding from the Geron Corporation. Private funding for experiments involving embryos was required because Congress attached a rider to legislation that affected FY1996 NIH funding. The rider, an amendment originally introduced by Representative Jay Dickey, prohibited HHS from using appropriated funds for the creation of human embryos for research purposes or for research in which human embryos are destroyed. The Dickey Amendment language has been added to each of the Labor, HHS, and Education appropriations acts for FY1997 through FY2008.[43] Funding for FY2009 is provided in the Omnibus Appropriations Act, 2009, P.L. 111-8 The Dickey Amendment is found in Section 509 of Division F— Departments of Labor, Health and Human Services, and Education, and Related Agencies Appropriations Act, 2009, of P.L. 111-8. It states that:

(a) None of the funds made available in this Act may be used for—
   the creation of a human embryo or embryos for research purposes; or

research in which a human embryo or embryos are destroyed, discarded,
or knowingly subjected to risk of injury or death greater than that
allowed for research on fetuses in utero under 45 CFR 46.204(b) and
Section 498(b) of the Public Health Service Act (42 U.S.C. 289g(b)).
For purposes of this section, the term 'human embryo or embryos' includes
any organism, not protected as a human subject under 45 CFR 46 [the
Human Subject Protection regulations] as of the date of enactment of this
Act, that is derived by fertilization, parthenogenesis, cloning, or any
other means from one or more human gametes [sperm or egg] or human
diploid cells [cells that have two sets of chromosomes, such as somatic
cells].

Clinton Administration Stem Cell Policy

Following the November 1998 announcement on the derivation of human
embryonic stem cells by scientists at the University of Wisconsin and Johns
Hopkins University, NIH requested a legal opinion from HHS on whether federal
funds could be used to support research on human stem cells derived from
embryos. The January 15, 1999, response from HHS General Counsel Harriet
Rabb found that the Dickey Amendment would not apply to research using
human stem cells "because such cells are not a human embryo within the statutory
definition." The finding was based, in part, on the determination by HHS that the
statutory ban on human embryo research defines an embryo as an *organism* that
when implanted in the uterus is capable of becoming a human being. Human stem
cells, HHS said, are not and cannot develop into an organism; they lack the
capacity to become organisms even if they are transferred to a uterus. As a result,
HHS maintained that NIH could support research that uses stem cells derived
through private funds, but could not support research that itself, with federal
funds, derives stem cells from embryos because of the federal ban in the Dickey
Amendment.

Shortly after the opinion by the HHS General Counsel was released, NIH
disclosed that the agency planned to fund research on stem cells derived from
human embryos once appropriate guidelines were developed and an oversight
committee established. NIH Director Harold Varmus appointed a working group
that began drafting guidelines in April 1999. Draft guidelines were published in
the *Federal Register* on December 2, 1999. About 50,000 comments were
received during the public comment period, which ended February 22, 2000. On

August 25, 2000, NIH published in the *Federal Register* final guidelines on the support of human embryonic stem cell research. The guidelines stated that studies utilizing "stem cells derived from human embryos may be conducted using NIH funds only if the cells were derived (without federal funds) from human embryos that were created for the purposes of fertility treatment and were in excess of the clinical need of the individuals seeking such treatment." Under the guidelines, NIH would not fund research directly involving the derivation of human stem cells from embryos; this was prohibited by the Dickey Amendment.

Other areas of research ineligible for NIH funding under the guidelines include (1) research in which human stem cells are utilized to create or contribute to a human embryo; (2) research in which human stem cells are combined with an animal embryo; (3) research in which human stem cells are used for reproductive cloning of a human; (4) research in which human stem cells are *derived* using somatic cell nuclear transfer (i.e., the transfer of a human somatic cell nucleus into a human or animal egg); (5) research *utilizing* human stem cells that were derived using somatic cell nuclear transfer; and (6) research utilizing stem cells that were derived from human embryos created for research purposes, rather than for infertility treatment.

NIH began accepting grant applications for research projects utilizing human stem cells immediately following publication of the guidelines; the deadline for submitting a grant application was March 15, 2001. All such applications were to be reviewed by the NIH Human Pluripotent Stem Cell Review Group (HPSCRG), which was established to ensure compliance with the guidelines. James Kushner, director of the University of Utah General Clinical Research Center, served briefly as chair of the HPSCRG. Applications would also have undergone the normal NIH peer-review process.[44] The first meeting of the HPSCRG was scheduled for April 25, 2001. The HPSCRG was to conduct an ethical review of human pluripotent stem cell lines to determine whether the research groups involved had followed the NIH guidelines in deriving the cell lines. However, in mid April 2001, HHS postponed the meeting until a review of the Clinton Administration's policy decisions on stem cell research was completed by the new administration following the election of George W. Bush.[45] According to media sources, the 12 HPSCRG members, whose names were not made public, represented a wide range of scientific, ethical and theological expertise and opinion, as well as at least one "mainstream Catholic."[46]

The Bush Administration conducted a legal review of the policy decisions made during the Clinton Administration regarding federal support of stem cell research, as well as a scientific review, prepared by NIH, of the status of the research and its applications. The scientific review was released on July 18, 2001, at a hearing on stem cell research held by the Senate Appropriations Subcommittee on Labor, Health and Human Services and Education.[47] The NIH report did not make any recommendations, but argued that both embryonic and adult stem cell research should be pursued.

George W. Bush Administration Stem Cell Policy

On August 9, 2001, President George W. Bush announced that for the first time federal funds would be used to support research on human embryonic stem cells, but funding would be limited to "existing stem cell lines where the life and death decision has already been made."[48] President Bush stated that the decision "allows us to explore the promise and potential of stem cell research without crossing a fundamental moral line, by providing taxpayer funding that would sanction or encourage further destruction of human embryos that have at least the potential for life." The President also stated that the federal government would continue to support research involving stem cells from other sources, such as umbilical cord blood, placentas, and adult and animal tissues, "which do not involve the same moral dilemma."

Under the Bush policy, federal funds may only be used for research on existing stem cell lines that were derived (1) with the informed consent of the donors, (2) from excess embryos created solely for reproductive purposes, and (3) without any financial inducements to the donors.[49] NIH was tasked with examining the derivation of all existing stem cell lines and creating a registry of those lines that satisfy the Bush Administration criteria. According to the White House, this will ensure that federal funds are used to support only stem cell research that is scientifically sound, legal, and ethical. Federal funds will not be used for (1) the derivation or use of stem cell lines derived from newly destroyed embryos, (2) the creation of any human embryos for research purposes, or (3) the cloning of human embryos for any purpose.

Impact of Bush Policy on Research

Over time, a growing number of scientists, disease advocates and others became concerned that federally supported research on human embryonic stem cells was limited to the number of cell lines that met the criteria of the August 9, 2001, Bush policy. Under the policy, only 21 cell lines were available for research with federal dollars. Because these pre-August 2001 cell lines were developed in the early days of human stem cell research using older 1990s techniques, the cell lines not only have the problems of xenotransplantion (described in the section below on FDA regulation), but they are harder to work with, are not as well characterized, and are genetically unstable compared to newer stem cell lines. In reaction to the limitations imposed by the Bush policy, several U.S. research groups decided to develop additional human embryonic stem cell lines using private funding or funds provided by state governments. In order to perform this work, the research groups were required to build new separate laboratories so that the group's federally funded research was conducted separately from research on the new stem cell lines.

A worldwide survey of laboratories conducted by the Boston Globe found that as of May 23, 2004, 128 human embryonic stem cell lines had been created since August 9, 2001; all were ineligible for use in federally funded research under the Bush policy on stem cell research.[50] Another survey of the number of human embryonic stem cell lines released in June 2006 found that as of January 1, 2006, 414 human embryonic stem cell lines had been created in at least 20 countries.[51]

Congressional Response to the Bush Policy

In response to concerns over access to human embryonic stem cell lines, in April 2004, a group of over 200 Members of the House of Representatives sent a letter to President George W. Bush requesting that the Administration revise the stem cell policy and utilize the embryos that are created in excess of need during the treatment of infertile couples.[52] The letter pointed out that an estimated 400,000 frozen IVF embryos[53] "will likely be destroyed if not donated, with informed consent of the couple, for research." According to the letter,

> scientists are reporting that it is increasingly difficult to attract new scientists to this area of research because of concerns that funding restrictions will keep this research from being successful. ... We have already seen researchers move to countries like the United Kingdom, which have more supportive policies. In addition, leadership in this area of research has shifted to the United Kingdom, which sees this scientific area as the cornerstone of its biotech industry.

Under the direction of the White House, then NIH Director Elias A. Zerhouni sent a letter in response to the House Members that restated the Bush Administration position against using federal funds for research involving the destruction of human embryos.[54] The letter from Dr. Zerhouni did contain the following sentence, which some observers believed in 2004 indicated a potential future policy shift: "And although it is fair to say that from a purely scientific perspective more cell lines may well speed some areas of human embryonic stem cell research, the president's position is still predicated on his belief that taxpayer funds should not 'sanction or encourage further destruction of human embryos that have at least the potential for life."[55] At the time, White House spokesperson Claire Buchan stated that the sentence did not indicate the president's position had changed. Supporters of stem cell research point out that the letter concedes that science could benefit from additional stem cell lines and that the president's position now rests solely on ethical arguments.

A letter signed by 58 Senators urging President Bush to expand the federal policy concerning embryonic stem cell research was sent on June 4, 2004.[56] The letter stated that "despite the fact that U.S. scientists were the first to derive human embryonic stem cells, leadership in this area of research is shifting to other countries such as the United Kingdom, Singapore, South Korea an dAustralia."[57]

On July 14, 2004, former HHS Secretary Tommy Thompson announced in a letter to then Speaker of the House Dennis Hastert that NIH would establish Centers of Excellence in Translational Stem Cell Research and a National Embryonic Stem Cell Bank.[58] The centers investigate how stem cells can be used to treat a variety of diseases and the bank collects in one location many of the stem cell lines that are eligible for federal research funding. In the letter to Speaker Hastert, Secretary Thompson stated that "before anyone can successfully argue the stem cell policy should be broadened, we must first exhaust the potential of the stem cell lines made available with the policy."[59] In reaction to the announcement, the President of the Coalition for the Advancement of Medical Research stated that "creating a bank to house stem cell lines created before August 2001 does nothing to increase the wholly inadequate supply of stem cell lines for research."[60] On October 3, 2005, NIH announced that it had awarded $16.1 million over four years to the WiCell Research Institute in Wisconsin to fund the National Stem Cell Bank.[61]

NIH also awarded $9.6 million over four years to fund two new Centers of Excellence in Translational Human Stem Cell Research, one at the University of California, Davis and the other at Northwestern University.

During the first session of the 109th Congress, the House passed H.R. 810 (Castle), the Stem Cell Research Enhancement Act of 2005, in May 2005. In July 2006, the Senate passed H.R. 810 and President George W. Bush immediately vetoed it, the first veto of his presidency. An attempt in the House to override the veto was unsuccessful.

During the 110th Congress, H.R. 3 (DeGette), the Stem Cell Research Enhancement Act of 2007, was introduced on January 5, 2007, with 211 cosponsors, and passed the House by a vote of 253 to 174 on January 11, 2007.[62] The Senate passed a companion bill, S. 5 (Reid), on April 11. 2007, by a vote of 63 to 34. The House passed S. 5 on June 7. 2007, by a vote of 247 to 176. President George W. Bush vetoed the bill on June 20, 2007, and signed Executive Order 13435, which directed the Secretary of HHS to "conduct and support research on the isolation, derivation, production and testing of stem cells that are capable of producing all or almost all of the cell types of the developing body and may result in improved understanding of or treatments for diseases and other adverse health conditions, but are derived without creating a human embryo for research purposes or destroying, discarding, or subjecting to harm a human embryo or fetus."[63] S. 5 was the same as H.R. 3, except it had an additional section supporting research on alternative human pluripotent stem cells.

Obama Administration Stem Cell Policy

On March 9, 2009, President Barack Obama signed an executive order revoking the Bush Presidential statement of August 9, 2001, as well as Executive Order 13435 signed by President Bush on June 20, 2007.[64] The Obama decision directs NIH to issue new guidelines for the conduct of human embryonic stem cell research within 120 days of the date of the executive order. NIH anticipates using some of the $10 billion in funds provided by the stimulus package (American Recovery and Reinvestment Act of 2009, P.L. 111-5) for research on human embryonic stem cells under the new guidelines.[65] The Obama decision will allow scientists to use federal funds for research utilizing the hundreds of human embryonic stem cell lines that have been created since the Bush 2001 policy. The International Society for Stem Cell Research estimates there are more than 800 such cell lines cited in the scientific literature, "but it is unclear how many to these lines would be eligible under the NIH guidelines."[66] The policy will also eliminate the need to separate federally funded research from research conducted with private funds on cell lines that were previously ineligible for federal funding under the Bush policy; this often required building new but duplicative laboratories under the Bush policy using funds that could have been spent on actual research.

On the same day, President Obama issued a memorandum on scientific integrity directing the head of the White House Office of Science and Technology Policy "to develop a strategy for restoring scientific integrity to government decision making."[67]

Stem Cell Research Regulation by Federal Agencies and Other Entities

The Common Rule (45 CFR 46, Subpart A) is a set of regulations that govern most federally funded research conducted on human beings. Its three basic requirements are aimed at protecting research subjects: the informed consent of research subjects, a review of proposed research by an Institutional Review Board (IRB), and institutional assurances of compliance with the regulations. However, ex vivo embryos (those not in a uterus) are not considered "human subjects" for these purposes, but federally funded research on human embryos is regulated by the Dickey Amendment as described above. Stem cells and stem cell lines are also not considered "human subjects," nor are they governed by the Dickey Amendment.

Because of the lack of federal regulation of stem cell research, the National Academies developed voluntary guidelines for deriving, handling and using human embryonic stem cells.[68] Two HHS agencies, FDA and NIH, regulate some aspects of stem cell research, even if research on stem cell lines is not classified as "human subjects" research. FDA, the agency that ensures the safety and efficacy of food, drugs, medical devices and cosmetics, regulates stem cell research aimed at the development of any "product" subject to its approval. NIH, the medical and behavioral research agency within HHS, regulates stem cell research that it funds in compliance with President Bush's 2001 policy. NIH has created a Human Embryonic Stem Cell Registry that lists the human embryonic stem cell lines that meet the eligibility criteria as outlined in the Bush Administration stem cell policy.

National Academies Guidelines

In July 2004 the National Academies established the committee on Guidelines for Human Embryonic Stem Cell Research to develop voluntary guidelines for deriving, handling and using human embryonic stem cells due to the current lack of federal regulation of such research. The stated position of the National Academies is that there should be a global ban on human reproductive cloning and therefore the guidelines will focus only on therapeutic and research uses of human embryonic stem cells and somatic cell nuclear transfer.

The committee released its "Guidelines for Human Embryonic Stem Cell Research" on April 26, 2005. The document provides guidance on informed consent of donors and states that there should be no financial incentives in the solicitation or donation of embryos, sperm, eggs, or somatic cells for research purposes. The guidelines recommend that each institution conducting human embryonic stem cell research establish an oversight committee, including experts in the relevant areas of science, ethics, and law, as well as members of the public, to review all proposed experiments. The guidelines recommend that a national panel be established to oversee the issue in general on a continuing basis.

The Human Embryonic Stem Cell Research Advisory Committee met for the first time in July 2006 and held a number of meetings to gather information about the need to revise the guidelines. In February 2007, a revised version of the guidelines was published with minor changes affecting Sections 1 (Introduction) and Section 2 (Establishment of an Institutional Embryonic Stem Cell Research Oversight Committee).[69] The guidelines were updated again in September 2008 to reflect the advances with iPS cells by including a new section entirely devoted to this new area of research.[70]

International Society for Stem Cell Research Guidelines

In February 2007, the International Society for Stem Cell Research (ISSCR) released its "Guidelines for the Conduct of Human Embryonic Stem Cell Research."[71] The ISSCR guidelines were developed by a committee of scientists, ethicists, and legal experts from 14 countries in order to "facilitate international collaboration by encouraging investigators and institutions to adhere to a uniform set of practices."[72] In drafting the guidelines, the ISSCR committee used as a model the National Academies guidelines, the regulations of the California Institute for Regenerative Medicine, and "governmental regulations already in place in other countries, particularly that of the Human Fertilisation and Embryology Authority of the United Kingdom."[73]

In order to ensure the responsible development of safe and effective stem cell therapies for patients, the ISSCR released in December 2008 a second guidance document, "Guidelines for the Clinical Translation of Stem Cells." In addition, due to concerns over unproven stem cell therapies being marketed directly to patients, the ISSCR also developed a handbook to be used by patients and their doctors in evaluating a stem cell therapy.[74] In the press release for the guidelines they noted "[t]oo often rogue clinics around the world exploit patients' hopes by offering unproven stem cell therapies, typically for large sums of money and without credible scientific rationale, oversight or patient protections."[75] According to ISSCR, this concern was substantiated by a study conducted by the University of Alberta, Canada, which analyzed the claims of 19 internet sites offering "stem cell therapies," the vast majority of which "over promise results and gravely underestimate the potential risks of their offered treatments."[76]

FDA Regulation

All of the human embryonic stem cell lines listed on the NIH Human Embryonic Stem Cell Registry (see **Table 2**) have been grown on beds of mouse "feeder" cells. The mouse cells secrete a substance that prevents the human embryonic stem cells from differentiating into more mature cell types (nerve or muscle cells). Infectious agents, such as viruses, within the mouse feeder cells could transfer into the human cells. If the human cells were transplanted into a patient, these infected human cells may cause disease in the patient which could be transmitted to close contacts of the patient and eventually to the general population. Public health officials and regulatory agencies such as the FDA are specifically concerned about retroviruses, which may remain hidden in the DNA only to cause disease many years later, as well as any unrecognized agents which may be present in the mouse cells.

The FDA defines "xenotransplantation" as "any procedure that involves the transplantation, implantation, or infusion into a human recipient of either (a) live cells, tissues, or organs from a nonhuman source, or (b) human body fluids, cells, tissues or organs that have had ex vivo contact with live nonhuman animal cells, tissues or organs."[77] Under FDA guidelines, transplantation therapy involving Bush approved stem cell lines, which all have been exposed to mouse feeder cells, would constitute xenotransplantation. Xenotransplantation products are subject to regulation by the FDA under Section 351 of the Public Health Service Act (42 USC 262) and the Federal Food, Drug and Cosmetic Act (21 USC 321 et seq.). FDA has developed guidance documents and the U.S. Public Health Service has developed guidelines on infectious disease issues associated with xenotransplantation.[78]

During a Senate hearing on stem cell research held by the Health, Education, Labor and Pensions Committee on September 5, 2001, the HHS Secretary stated that the FDA was overseeing 17 investigational protocols involving xenotransplantation in other areas of clinical research that involve patients. Therefore, he said, the xenotransplantation-related public health concerns over the human embryonic stem cell lines may not necessarily preclude the development of treatments for patients. While the problems presented by xenotransplantation for clinical research are neither unique to stem cell research nor insurmountable, many scientists believe it will be preferable to use sterile cell lines when attempting to treat patients via stem cell transplantation, and scientists have been successful in developing human embryonic stem cells that can be maintained without the use of mouse feeder cells.[79]

Table 1. National Institutes of Health Funding ($ in millions)

Stem Cell Research	FY04	FY05	FY06	FY07	FY08
Human Embryonic	24	40	38	74	88
Non-Human Embryonic	89	97	110	120	150
Human Non-Embryonic	203	199	206	226	297
Non-Human Non-Embryonic	236	273	289	400	497
Human Cord Blood/Placenta	16	15	16	38	38
Non-Human Cord Blood/Placenta	3	3	4	9	9
Total, Stem Cell Research	**553**	**609**	**643**	**968**	**938**

Source: NIH website, January 15, 2009, http://report.nih.gov/rcdc/categories/ PFSummaryTable.aspx.

NIH Research Funding and Stem Cell Registry under the Bush Policy

The August 9, 2001, Bush Administration policy statement on stem cell research and the NIH Stem Cell Registry effectively replaced the NIH stem cell guidelines that were developed under the Clinton Administration and never fully implemented. Grant proposals for embryonic stem cell research underwent only the normal peer-review process without the added review of the HPSCRG as had been specified under the Clinton NIH stem cell guidelines. In February 2002, NIH announced the approval of the first expenditures for research on human embryonic stem cells. Funding for stem cell research by NIH is shown in **Table 1**. The NIH website provides additional information about stem cell activities and funding opportunities.[80]

The NIH Human Embryonic Stem Cell Registry lists stem cell lines that were eligible for use in federally funded research under the Bush policy.[81] As shown in **Table 2**, the NIH registry originally listed universities and companies that had derived a total of 78 human embryonic stem cell lines which were eligible for use in federally funded research under the August 2001 Bush Administration policy. However, many of these stem cell lines were found to be either unavailable or unsuitable for research. As of May 4, 2007, the NIH registry listed a total of 21 stem cell lines available from six sources.

Table 2. NIH List of Human Embryonic Stem Cell Lines Eligible for Use in Federal Research

Namea	Number of stem cell lines	
	Eligible	Available
BresaGen, Inc., Athens, GA	4	3
Cell & Gene Therapy Institute (Pochon CHA University), Seoul, Korea	2	
Cellartis AB, Goteborg, Sweden	3	2
CyThera, Inc., San Diego, CA	9	0
ES Cell International, Melbourne, Australia	6	6
Geron Corporation, Menlo Park, CA	7	
Goteborg University, Goteborg, Sweden	16	
Karolinska Institute, Stockholm, Sweden	6	0
Maria Biotech Co. Ltd.—Maria Infertility Hospital Medical Institute, Seoul, Korea	3	
MizMedi Hospital—Seoul National University, Seoul, Korea	1	0
National Center for Biological Sciences/Tata Institute of Fundamental Research,		
Bangalore, India	3	
Reliance Life Sciences, Mumbai, India	7	
Technion University, Haifa, Israel	4	3
University of California, San Francisco, CA	2	2
Wisconsin Alumni Research Foundation, Madison, WI	5	5
Total	78	21

Source: NIH website, February 3, 2009,
     http://stemcells.nih.gov/research/registry/eligibilityCriteria.asp.
     a. Six table entries do not have stem cell lines available for shipment to U.S. researchers because of a variety of scientific, regulatory and legal reasons. The zeros entered in the "Available" column indicate that "the cells failed to expand into undifferentiated cell cultures."

State Laws that Restrict Stem Cell Research[82]

Many states restrict research on aborted fetuses or embryos, but research is often permitted with consent of the parent or parents. Almost half of the states also restrict the sale of fetuses or embryos. Louisiana is the only state that specifically prohibits research on in vitro fertilized (IVF) embryos. Illinois and Michigan also prohibit research on live embryos. Arkansas, Indiana, Michigan, North Dakota and South Dakota prohibit research on cloned embryos. Virginia may also ban research on cloned embryos, but the statute may leave room for interpretation because human being is not defined. (There may be disagreement about whether human being includes blastocysts, embryos or fetuses.) California, Connecticut, Illinois, Iowa, Massachusetts, New Jersey, New York, and Rhode Island have laws that prohibit cloning for the purpose of initiating a pregnancy, but allow cloning for research.

Several states limit the use of state funds for cloning or stem cell research. Missouri forbids the use of state funds for reproductive cloning but not for cloning for the purpose of stem cell research, and Maryland's statutes prohibit state-funded stem cell researchers from engaging in reproductive cloning. Arizona law prohibits the use of public monies for reproductive or therapeutic cloning. Nebraska statutes limit the use of state funds for embryonic stem cell research. Restrictions only apply to state healthcare cash funds provided by tobacco settlement dollars. State funding available under Illinois Executive Order 6 (2005) may not be used for reproductive cloning or for research on fetuses from induced abortions.

Despite restrictive federal and state policies, several states (California, Connecticut, Illinois, Indiana, Maryland, Massachusetts, New Jersey, New York, Ohio, Washington, Wisconsin, Virginia) are encouraging or providing funding for stem cell research (adult, embryonic, and in some cases SCNT as well), as they seek to remain competitive and prevent the relocation of scientists and biotechnology firms to other states or overseas.

Legislation in the 111ᵗʰ Congress

H.R. 873 (DeGette), the Stem Cell Research Enhancement Act of 2009, was introduced on February 4, 2009. The text of H.R. 873 is identical to legislation introduced in the 110ᵗʰ Congress, H.R. 3 (DeGette), and the 109ᵗʰ Congress, H.R.

810 (Castle). The bill would allow federal support for research that utilizes human embryonic stem cells regardless of the date on which the stem cells were derived from a human embryo, and thus if passed would negate the August 2001 Bush stem cell policy limitation. It would amend the Public Health Service (PHS) Act by adding a new Section 498D, "Human Embryonic Stem Cell Research." The new section would direct the Secretary of HHS to conduct and support research that utilizes human embryonic stem cells regardless of the date on which the stem cells were derived from a human embryo. Stem cell lines must meet ethical guidelines established by the NIH. In order to be eligible for federal research, stem cell lines must have be derived from embryos that were originally created for fertility treatment purposes and were in excess of clinical need. In addition, only embryos that the individuals seeking fertility treatments had determined would not be implanted in a woman, and would be discarded, would be eligible for stem cell derivation. Written consent would be required for embryo donation. The Secretary, in consultation with the Director of NIH, would promulgate guidelines 60 days after enactment. No federal funds would be used to conduct research on unapproved stem cell lines. The Secretary would annually report to Congress about stem cell research.

H.R. 872 (DeGette), the Stem Cell Research Improvement Act of 2009, was also introduced on February 4, 2009. It is similar to H.R. 873 in that it adds the same Section 498D, "Human Embryonic Stem Cell Research," to the PHS Act, but it also adds another Section 498E, "Guidelines on Research Involving Human Stem Cells," which would require the Director of NIH to issue guidelines on research involving human embryonic stem cell within 90 days of enactment; updates of the guidelines would be required every three years.

S. 487 (Harkin), the Stem Cell Research Enhancement Act of 2009, was introduced on February 26, 2009. S. 487 is the same as H.R. 873, except it has an additional section supporting research on alternative human pluripotent stem cells.[83] This section would amend the Public Health Service Act by adding a new Section 498E, "Alternative Human Pluripotent Stem Cell Research." The new section would require the Secretary of HHS to develop techniques for the isolation, derivation, production, and testing of stem cells that are capable of producing all or almost all of the cell types of a developing body, and may result in improved understanding of treatments for diseases, but that are not derived from a human embryo. The Secretary, after consulting with the Director of NIH, would be required to (1) provide guidance concerning the next steps for additional research, (2) prioritize research that holds the greatest potential for near-term clinical benefit, and (3) take into account techniques outlined by the

President's Council on Bioethics and any other appropriate techniques and research. The Secretary would be required to prepare and submit to the appropriate committees of Congress an annual report describing the activities and research conducted. S. 487 would authorize such sums as may be necessary for FY2010 through FY2012. The bill is identical to a bill in the 110th Congress, S. 5 (Reid), which passed the Senate and House and was vetoed by President Bush in June 2007.

End Notes

[1] "Removing Barriers to Responsible Scientific Research Involving Human Stem Cells," March 9, 2009, at [http://www.whitehouse.gov/the_press_office/Removing-Barriers-to-Responsible-Scientific-Research-Involving- Human-Stem-Cells/].

[2] "Obama Signs Executive Order Reversing Bush's Embryonic Stem Cell Research Policy," *Health Care Daily Report*, March 10, 2009.

[3] The White House, Office of the Press Secretary, Remarks of President Barack Obama-As Prepared for Delivery, Signing of Stem Cell Executive Order and Scientific Integrity Presidential Memorandum, March 9, 2009, at [http://www.whitehouse.gov/the_press_office/Remarks-of-the-President-As-Prepared-for-Delivery-Signing-of-Stem-Cell-Executive-Order-and-Scientific-Integrity-Presidential-Memorandum/].

[4] Alex Wayne, "With Obama Reversal of Stem Cell Policy, Democrats Look to Expand Funding," *CQ Today*, March 9, 2009.

[5] For further information, see CRS Report RL33554, *Stem Cell Research: Ethical Issues*, by Erin D. Williams and Judith A. Johnson.

[6] Drew Armstrong, "NIH Chief's Opinion on Stem Cell Research Goes Afield of White House Policy," *CQ Today*, March 19, 2007.

[7] Ibid.

[8] John Reichard, "Zerhouni Makes Strong Case Against Bush Policy on Stem Cells, NIH Funding," *CQ Today*, March 19, 2005.

[9] An archived audio webcast of the May 8, 2008, hearing can be found athttp://energycommerce.house.gov/ cmte_mtgs/110-he-hrg.050808.StcmCcll.shtml.

[10] During the first session of the 109th Congress, the House passed identical legislation, H.R. 810 (Castle), in May 2005. In July 2006, the Senate passed H.R. 810 and President Bush immediately vetoed it, the first veto of his presidency. An attempt in the House to override the veto was unsuccessful.

[11] A pluripotent cell has the ability to differentiate into all of the various cell types that make up the body, but not the "extra-embryonic" tissues such as the components of the placenta.

[12] The IVF embryos were originally created for the treatment of infertility. Excess embryos are often frozen for future use. A couple may elect to discard their excess embryos, donate the embryos for research, or allow another couple to adopt an embryo. The Society for Assisted Reproductive Technology and RAND conducted a survey of more than 430 infertility clinics to determine the number of frozen embryos in the United States; 340 clinics responded to the survey. Nearly 400,000 embryos have been frozen and stored since the late 1970s. The vast majority of embryos are being held to help couples have children at a later date. Patients have

designated 2.8%, or about 11,000 embryos, for research. Scientists estimate these 11,000 could form up to 275 stem cell lines, perhaps much less http://www.rand.org/pubs/research_briefs/RB9038/index1.html.

[13] Scientists and physicians use the term "embryo" for the first eight weeks after fertilization, and "fetus" for the ninth week through birth. In contrast, the Department of Health and Human Services (HHS) regulations define "fetus" as "the product of conception from the time of implantation" (45 C.F.R. § 46.203).

[14] Gretchen Vogel and Constance Holden, "Field Leaps Forward with New Stem Cell Advances," *Science*, v. 318, November 23, 2007, pp. 1224-1225.

[15] Dennis Normile, "Shinya Yamanaka: Modest Researcher, Results to Brag About," *Science*, v. 319, February 1, 2008, p. 562.

[16] Constance Holden and Gretchen Vogel, "A Seismic Shift for Stem Cell Research," *Science*, v. 319, February 1, 2008, pp. 560-563.

[17] A somatic cell is a body cell. In contrast, a germ cell is an egg or sperm cell.

[18] Dolly was euthanized in February 2003 after developing a lung infection. Some claim her death at six years was related to being a clone, but her ailment may also have occurred because she was raised indoors (for security reasons) rather than as a pastured sheep, which often live to 12 years of age. G. Kolata, "First Mammal Clone Dies," *New York Times*, February 15, 2003, p. A4.

[19] Elizabeth Finkel, "Researchers Derive Stem Cells From Monkeys," *ScienceNOW Daily News*, June 19, 2007.

[20] Vogel and Holden, "Field Leaps Forward with New Stem Cell Advances," p. 1224.

[21] For further information, see CRS Report RL31358, *Human Cloning*, by Judith A. Johnson and Erin D. Williams.

[22] Gretchen Vogel, "Collaborators Split over Ethics Allegations" *Science*, November 18, 2005, p. 1100.

[23] Nicholas Wade and Choe Sang-Hun, "Researcher Faked Evidence of Human Cloning, Koreans Report," *The New York Times*, January 10, 2006, p. A1.

[24] Dennis Normile, Gretchen Vogel, and Constance Holden, "Cloning Researcher Says Work is Flawed but Claims Results Stand," *Science*, December 23, 2005, p. 1886-1887; Carl T. Hall, "UCSF Resumes Human Embryo Stem Cell Work," *The San Francisco Chronicle*, May 6, 2006, p. A.1.

[25] Julio C. Voltarelli, et al., "Autologous Nonmyeloablative Hematopoietic Stem Cell Transplantation in Newly Diagnosed Type 1 Diabetes Mellitus," *Journal of the American Medical Association*, April 11, 2007, v. 297, p. 1568-1576.

[26] Comments made by NIH Director Elias Zerhouni during a May 8, 2008 hearing before the House Energy and Commerce Subcommittee on Health, audio webcast available at http://energycommerce.house.gov/ cmte_mtgs/110-he-hrg.050808.StemCell.shtml.

[27] Rick Weiss, "Scientists See Potential in Amniotic Stem Cells; They Are Highly Versatile And Readily Available," *The Washington Post*, January 8, 2007, p. A1, A5.

[28] Frederick R. Appelbaum, "Hematopoietic-Cell Transplantation at 50," *The New England Journal of Medicine*, v. 357, October 11, 2007, pp. 1472-1475.

[29] http://www.stemcellresearch.org/facts/treatments.htm.

[30] Shane Smith, William Neaves and Steven Teitelbaum, "Adult Stem Cell Treatments for Diseases?"*Science*, v. 313, July 28, 2006, p. 439; as well as online in *Sciencexpress*, July 13, 2006, p. 1 http://www.sciencexpress.org.

[31] David A. Prentice and Gene Tarne, "Treating Diseases with Adult Stem Cells," *Science*, v. 315, January 19, 2007, p. 328.

[32] Shane Smith, William Neaves and Steven Teitelbaum, "Adult Versus Embryonic Stem Cells: Treatments," *Science*, v. 316, June 8, 2007, p. 1422.

[33] David A. Prentice and Gene Tarne, "Adult Versus Embryonic Stem Cells: Treatments—Response," *Science*, v. 316, June 8, 2007, p. 1422-1423.

[34] National Institutes of Health, Department of Health and Human Services, *Stem Cells: Scientific Progress and Future Research Directions*, June 2001, available at http://stemcells.nih.gov/info/scireport/. Institute of Medicine, *Stem Cells and the Future of Regenerative Medicine*, 2002, available at http://www.nas.edu.

[35] Andrew Pollack, "FDA approves a stem cell trial," *New York Times*, January 23, 2009.

[36] Ibid.

[37] Jennifer Couzin, "Celebration and concern over U.S. trial of embryonic stem cells," *Science*, vol. 323 (January 30, 2009), p. 568.

[38] Chimeras have been created by scientists in a variety of different ways and have been the subject of research studies for many years. Human chimeras occur naturally when two eggs become fertilized and, instead of developing into twins, they fuse in the uterus creating a single embryo with two distinct sets of genes. For one example, see Constance Holden, "Chimera on a Bike?" *Science*, June 24, 2005, p. 1864.

[39] The EAB was created in 1978 by the Department of Health Education and Welfare (HEW), the forerunner of the Department of Health and Human Services (HHS). The EAB was formed at the recommendation of the National Commission for the Protection of Human Subjects of Biomedical and Behavioral Research. The National Commission operated from 1974 to 1978 and issued 10 reports, many of which formed the basis of federal regulations for research involving human subjects (45 C.F.R. Part 46).

[40] These were *blastomere separation*, where a two- to eight-cell embryo is treated causing the cells (blastomeres) to separate, and *blastocyst division*, in which an embryo at the more advanced blastocyst stage is split into two.

[41] National Institutes of Health, *Report of the Human Embryo Research Panel*, Sept. 27, 1994.

[42] However, federal funds have been provided for research on both human and animal adult stem cells and animal embryonic stem cells.

[43] The rider language has not changed significantly from year to year (however there was a technical correction in P.L. 109-149). The original rider can be found in Section 128 of P.L. 104-99; it affected NIH funding for FY1996 contained in P.L. 104-91. For subsequent fiscal years, the rider is found in Title V, General Provisions, of the Labor, HHS and Education appropriations acts in the following public laws: FY1997, P.L. 104-208; FY1998, P.L. 105-78; FY1999, P.L. 105-277; FY2000, P.L. 106-113; FY2001, P.L. 106-554; FY2002, P.L. 107-116; FY2003, P.L. 108-7; FY2004, P.L. 108-199; FY2005, P.L. 108-447; FY2006, P.L. 109-149; FY2007, P.L. 110-5; FY2008, P.L. 110-161.

[44] According to media sources, as of April 2001 only three grant applications had been submitted to NIH, and one was subsequently withdrawn. (*Washington FAX*, April 19, 2001.) Presumably, scientists were reluctant to invest the time and effort into preparing the necessary paperwork for the NIH grant application process when the prospects of receiving federal funding were uncertain under the new Bush Administration. (P. Recer, "Stem Cell Studies Said Hurt by Doubt," *AP Online*, May 2, 2001.) In a related development, one of the leading U.S. researchers on stem cells, Roger Pederson of the University of California, San Francisco, decided to move his laboratory to the United Kingdom for "the possibility of carrying out my research with human embryonic stem cells with public support." (Aaron Zitner, "Uncertainty Is Thwarting Stem Cell Researchers," *Los Angeles Times*, July 16, 2001, pp. A1, A8.) Human embryonic stem cell research was approved overwhelmingly by the House of Commons in December 2000 and the House of Lords in January 2001.

[45] Rick Weiss, "Bush Administration Order Halts Stem Cell Meeting; NIH Planned Session to Review Fund Requests," *Washington Post*, April 21, 2001, p. A2.

[46] Ibid.

[47] National Institutes of Health, Department of Health and Human Services. *Stem Cells: Scientific Progress and Future Research Directions*, June 2001. The NIH scientific report can be found at http://stemcells.nih.gov/info/scireport/.

[48] The August 9, 2001, *Remarks by the President on Stem Cell Research* can be found http://georgewbushwhitehouse.archives.gov/news/releases/2001/08/20010809-2.html

[49] The White House, *Fact Sheet on Embryonic Stem Cell Research*, August 9, 2001, found at http://georgewbushwhitehouse.archives.gov/news/releases/2001/08/20010809-1.html

[50] Gareth Cook, "94 New Cell Lines Created Abroad since Bush Decision," *Boston Globe*, May 23, 2004, p. A14.

[51] Anke Guhr, et al., "Current State of Human Embryonic Stem Cell Research: An Overview of Cell Lines and Their Use in Experimental Work," *Stem Cells 2006*, v. 24, p. 2187-2191, found at http://www.StemCells.com.

[52] See http://www.house.gov/degette/news/releases/040428.pdf.

[53] A survey conducted in 2002 and published in 2003 by the Society for Assisted Reproductive Technology and RAND determined that nearly 400,000 frozen embryos are stored in the United States, but most are currently targeted for patient use. See David I. Hoffman et al., "Cryopreserved Embryos in the United States and Their Availability for Research," *Fertility and Sterility*, vol. 79, May 2003, pp. 1063-1069.

[54] Rick Weiss, "Bush's Stem Cell Policy Reiterated, but Some See Shift," *The Washington Post*, May 16, 2004, p. A18.

[55] Letter from Elias A. Zerhouni, Director, National Institutes of Health, to The Honorable Diana DeGette and The Honorable Michael Castle, May 14, 2004.

[56] See http://feinstein.senate.gov/04Releases/r-stemcell-ltr.pdf.

[57] Ibid.

[58] Andrew J. Hawkins, "NIH Stem Cell Bank, Centers of Excellence Will Fast-Track Translational Research, Says Thompson," *Washington FAX*, July 15, 2004.

[59] Ibid.

[60] Ibid.

[61] NIH Press Office, "NIH Awards a National Stem Cell Bank and New Centers of Excellence in Translational Human Stem Cell Research," October 3, 2005, http://www.nih.gov/news/pr/oct2005/od-03.htm. The website for WiCell and the National Stem Cell Bank can be found at http://www.wicell.org/.

[62] During the first session of the 109th Congress, the House passed identical legislation, H.R. 810 (Castle), in May 2005. In July 2006, the Senate passed H.R. 810 and President Bush immediately vetoed it, the first veto of his presidency. An attempt in the House to override the veto was unsuccessful.

[63] The White House, Office of the Press Secretary, "Executive Order: Expanding Approved Stem Cell Lines in Ethically Responsible Ways," June 20, 2007, found at http://georgewbushwhitehouse.archives.gov/ news/releases/2007/06/20070620-6.html

[64] "Removing Barriers to Responsible Scientific Research Involving Human Stem Cells," March 9, 2009, at [http://www.whitehouse.gov/the_press_office/Removing-Barriers-to-Responsible-Scientific-Research-Involving- Human-Stem-Cells/].

[65] "Obama Signs Executive Order Reversing Bush's Embryonic Stem Cell Research Policy," *Health Care Daily Report*, March 10, 2009.

[66] Ibid.

[67] The White House, Office of the Press Secretary, Remarks of President Barack Obama-As Prepared for Delivery, Signing of Stem Cell Executive Order and Scientific Integrity Presidential Memorandum, March 9, 2009, at [http://www.whitehouse.gov/the_press_office/Remarks-of-

the-President-As-Prepared-for-Delivery-Signing-of-Stem-Cell-Executive-Order-and-Scientific-Integrity-Presidential-Memorandum/].

[68] The National Academies bring together committees of experts in all areas of science and technology to address critical national issues and give advice on a pro bono basis to the federal government and the public. The National Academies is comprised of four organizations: the National Academy of Sciences (NAS), established by Abraham Lincoln in 1863; the National Academy of Engineering, established by NAS in 1964; the Institute of Medicine, established by NAS in 1970; and, the National Research Council, established in 1916 by NAS at the request of President Wilson.

[69] The 2007 Amendment to the 2005 Guidelines for Human Embryonic Stem Cell Research can be found at http://www.nap.edu/catalog/11278.html.

[70] The original 2005 Guidelines as well as the 2007 amended version and the 2008 amended version can be found at http://www.nap.edu/catalog.php?record_id=12553.

[71] The ISSCR Guidelines can be found at http://www.isscr.org/guidelines/index.htm.

[72] George Q. Daley, Lars Ahrlund-Richter, and Jonathan M. Auerbach, et al., "The ISSCR Guidelines for Human Embryonic Stem Cell Research," *Science*, vol. 315 (February 2, 2007), pp. 603-604.

[73] Ibid.

[74] The ISSCR Guidelines and the Patient Handbook are at http://www.isscr.org/clinical_trans/index.cfm.

[75] International Society for Stem Cell Research, "The ISSCR Releases New Guidelines to Shape Future of Stem Cell Therapy," press release, December 3, 2008, http://www.isscr.org/press_releases/clinicalguidelines.html.

[76] Ibid.

[77] Xenotransplantation Action Plan: FDA approach to the regulation of xenotransplantation. Available at http://www.fda.gov/cber/xap/xap.htm.

[78] These documents are available at http://www.fda.gov/cber/xap/xap.htm.

[79] National Institutes of Health, Department of Health and Human Services, *Stem Cells: Scientific Progress and Future Research Directions*, June 2001, pp. 95-96; Susanne Rust, "UW Grows Animal-Free Stem Cell Lines," *The Milwaukee Journal Sentinel*, January 2, 2006, p. A1.

[80] See http://stemcells.nih.gov/research/funding/.

[81] Information about the NIH Human Embryonic Stem Cell Registry iavailable at http://stemcells.nih.gov/research/registry/index.asp.

[82] The information in this section was obtained from "State Embryonic and Fetal Research Laws," updated January 2008 on the National Council of State Legislatures website, at http://www.ncsl.org/programs/health/genetics/embfet.htm, visited February 3, 2009.

[83] A pluripotent cell has the ability to differentiate into all of the various cell types that make up the body, but not the "extra-embryonic" tissues such as the components of the placenta.

In: Stem Cell Research and Science
Editor: Brenden E. Aylesworth

ISBN: 978-1-60876-083-1
© 2010 Nova Science Publishers, Inc.

Chapter 4

Testimony to be Presented to the House Committee on Energy and Commerce's Subcommittee on Health by Joseph R. Bertino

Joseph R. Bertino

Good Morning, Mr. Chairman, Members of the Committee. Thank you for inviting me to present my testimony today.

"Stem Cells" are defined as cells capable of self-renewal as well as differentiation. The investigators funded by the New Jersey State Commission on Science are exploring every type of stem cell for the purpose of understanding function, regulation, and potential therapeutic benefit. These studies range from very basic studies to studies that will soon be translated into the clinic.

The promise of stem cell research is compelling and far-reaching. No other line of scientific inquiry offers better hope for curing intractable medical conditions. Indeed, therapies based on stem cells are a paradigm shift in the modern medical revolution. The potential to treat currently incurable conditions is both real and achievable in our lifetimes.

As a society, we have an obligation to pursue scientific discoveries that offer a clear potential to help those living with devastating illnesses. At the same, we recognize the legitimate moral, social and religious concerns raised by new technologies.

To address such concerns, nationally respected science associations, federal agencies and the State of New Jersey have set forth policies and procedures that ensure stem cell research meets the highest scientific and ethical standards. The Stem Cell Institute of New Jersey is committed to conducting responsible research that complies fully with these stringent requirements.

History of Stem Cell Research in New Jersey

On May 12, 2004, the Stem Cell Institute of New Jersey was created by a memorandum of understanding between Rutgers, the State University of New Jersey and UMDNJ-Robert Wood Johnson Medical School.

The State committed $8.5 million in state funds to support work at the Stem Cell Institute in financial year 2006, including $5.5 million in capital funds to Robert Wood Johnson Medical School and Rutgers University to support laboratory renovation and GMP facilities to support stem cell research, as well as two clinical trials using umbilical cord-derived stem cells.

In December 2005, NJ became the first state to finance research using human embryonic stem cells. The Commission on Science and Technology awarded a total of $5 million to 17 research teams.

On October 19, 2006, the finance committee of the General Assembly passed a $250 million bill to support stem cell research facilities in New Brunswick, Camden, and Newark.

In October 2006, monthly meetings of investigators interested in stem cell research were initiated at Rutgers and Robert Wood Johnson Medical School. Over fifty investigators from academic and pharmaceutical companies have been meeting to report their work in stem cell research, to discuss progress in the field and to plan collaborative experiments.

In 2007, New Jersey awarded 17 grants, totaling $10 million to stem cell researchers, including two grants to fund core laboratories for embryonic stem cell research.

Despite polls that showed that the majority of New Jerseyans were in favor of supporting embryonic stem cell research, a referendum was defeated in November 2007 that would have provided $450 million dollars, for ten years in support of stem cell research. Major reasons for the defeat of the referendum were the off-year election, with fewer than 30% of voters coming to the polls, and the concern that this would add to the public's tax burden, as well as put New Jersey even further in the red.

Governor Corzine continues to be a strong supporter of stem cell research and the building of the joint Rutgers/UMDNJ-RWJMS Stem Cell Institute in New Brunswick. Key members of the NJ legislature also continue to strongly support stem cell research.

In June 2008, an additional 10 million dollars will be made available for investigators in New Jersey from the State for stem cell research via a peer-reviewed grant program.

Examples of studies in progress are as follows below

Two types of stem cells are found in the bone marrow: hematopoetic stem cells, that form blood cells, and mesenchymal stem cells, capable of differentiating or forming bone, cartilage, nerve cells, fat cells, etc. Hematopoeitic stem cells are now used at the RWJUH and throughout the world to treat patients with cancer following chemotherapy. Mesenchymal stem cells from bone marrow or cord blood are being tested for their ability to prevent graft vs. host disease, after marrow transplantation. Other uses for mesenchymal stem cells under study by NJ investigators include targeting tumors with mesenchymal stem cells carrying toxins, and use in regenerative medicine (spinal cord injury, heart injury and brain disorders (Parkinson's, Alzheimer's)).

Researchers at both Rutgers and UMDNJ have special expertise and interest in neural stem cells that may have important implications for brain disorders as well as serve as models to promote drug discovery.

Cord blood, placenta and amniotic fluid are also a rich source of stem cells. Clinical trials are in progress in collaboration with investigators in China, using a subset of these cells to treat spinal cord injury (Dr. Wise Young). The characterization of stem cells from placenta is under study by RJWMS investigators in collaboration with Celgene, a NJ-based biotech company.

Work on human embryonic stem cells has been hampered by Federal guidelines that limit studies to 20 cell lines that have been around for several years. The two core laboratories at Rutgers and RWJMS, established with NJ State funding, have allowed investigators to expand research activities using newly established embryonic cell lines.

Importantly, the completion of a GMP facility at the Cancer Institute/Stem Cell Institute will allow stem cells to be produced in quantities necessary for clinical studies.

The funding provided by the State of New Jersey has provided key support for both the research outlined above and additional research programs focused on a variety of important disease conditions including multiple sclerosis, Parkinson's disease, Alzheimer's disease and diabetes. A key part of our efforts has been the establishment of stem cell banking of umbilical cord blood and other stem cells. New Jersey's stem cell banks are leaders in this field.

I would be happy to answer the committee's questions. Thank you.

In: Stem Cell Research and Science
Editor: Brenden E. Aylesworth

ISBN: 978-1-60876-083-1
© 2010 Nova Science Publishers, Inc.

Chapter 5

Testimony to House Committee on Energy and Commerce, Subcommittee on Health "Stem Cell Science: The Foundation for Future Cures"

George Q. Daley

Thank you for the invitation to speak today on the subject of stem cell science. My name is George Daley and I am an Associate Professor of Biological Chemistry, Medicine, and Pediatrics at Children's Hospital Boston and Harvard Medical School, a core faculty member of the Harvard Stem Cell Institute, an investigator of the Howard Hughes Medical Institute, and the current President of the International Society for Stem Cell Research (ISSCR), the major professional organization of stem cell scientists worldwide. My laboratory studies blood development, blood cancer, and experimental transplant therapies for diseases like sickle cell anemia, immune deficiency and leukemia. In my clinical duties at Children's Hospital, I care for patients with these devastating blood diseases, and see first hand the need for better treatments. Stem cell research offers hope.

Let me recount the stories of two patients I cared for recently at Children's Hospital that illustrate the shortcomings of current therapies. One was a young African-American boy with sickle cell anemia, suddenly struck down by what we call a pain crisis. When I saw him in the emergency room, he was writhing on the gurney, and whimpering in pain. Despite powerful, high doses of intravenous morphine, I was unable to give that child adequate relief from his pain and suffering for several days. A second case was an infant who suffered repeated infections and had spent half his young life in the hospital hooked up to intravenous antibiotics. His disease was immune-deficiency, and unfortunately he had no sibling donors for a potentially curative adult stem cell transplant. Stem cell research is laying the foundation for improved treatments for these kids, and countless other children and adults with debilitating, life-threatening diseases.

All stem cells—whether from embryonic, fetal, neonatal, or adult sources—hold great promise. The crowning scientific achievement of the twentieth century was the sequencing of the human genome, and the dominant mission of twenty-first century science is to discover how that blueprint drives the formation of tissues and organs, and how tissues are sustained, repaired, and rejuvenated over time. Stem cell research goes to the core of human biology and medicine.

Much excitement in stem cell research has focused on a property of embryonic cells called pluripotency—the capacity to generate all of the tissues in an organism. Recently, several laboratories, including my own, reported that a small set of genes linked to pluripotency in embryonic stem (ES) cells can be inserted into human skin cells to induce pluripotency—to endow skin cells with this same remarkable capacity to become a seed for all tissues in the body. By using gene-based reprogramming to make these so-called induced pluripotent stem cells (called "iPS cells"), scientists can now produce customized, patient-specific stem cells in the Petri dish. In a matter of weeks, we can take cells from a patient's forearm and transform them into pluripotent stem cells that we believe closely approximate embryonic stem cells. This is a major breakthrough in medical research, empowering scientists to create cellular models of human disease. It may also mean that one day we will treat patients with rejuvenated and repaired versions of their own tissues.

Realizing this promise will take time. A key concern is that the viruses used to carry the reprogramming genes into human skin cells can cause cancer. Moreover, the genes and pathways the viruses stimulate are themselves associated with cancer, raising the concern that even if viruses can be eliminated from the process, the reprogrammed cells might remain predisposed to cancer. For these reasons, iPS cells may never be suitable for use in patients. I sincerely hope that iPS cells are the long-sought-after customized patient-specific stem cell, but much more research must be done.

Even with iPS cells in hand, my laboratory will continue to study embryonic stem cells. First, we need to directly compare the capacity of these two types of stem cells to generate specific tissues. Some very preliminary data has suggested that iPS cells may be less potent than embryonic stem cells in making blood, while others are noting a deficiency in making heart muscle cells. It will take years for scientists to understand the similarities and differences between these two valuable classes of pluripotent stem cells. Even with iPS cells in hand, my laboratory will continue to investigate somatic cell nuclear transfer as a means of generating pluripotent stem cells. Reprogramming by nuclear transfer is faster and may entail very different mechanisms than gene-based reprogramming. Learning why may lead to better methods for making iPS cells.

The iPS breakthrough is being heralded by opponents of embryonic stem cell research as a solution to the long-smoldering debate over the necessity of embryonic stem cell research. We have heard the arguments for many years, first made when multi-potential adult progenitor cells (MAPCs) were reported in 2002, and later when stem cells were isolated from Fat and Amniotic fluid: we are told that alternatives are available that preclude the need for embryonic stem cell research. Congress has been wise to not yield to such arguments. Indeed, it was embryonic stem cell research that led directly to the breakthrough in iPS cells, and my own laboratory was poised to generate iPS cells in large part because of our experience and expertise in deriving and culturing human embryonic stem cells. Today, it would again be a mistake to place limits on the tools available to biomedical scientists to pursue the next medical breakthroughs. The right course for biomedical science and ultimately the right decision for patients and our health care system, is to expand the scope of federal funding for all forms of stem cell research, including the many lines of embryonic stem cells created after the President's artificial deadline of August 9th, 2001.

Yesterday, in my address to the Congressional Biomedical Research Caucus, I was asked the question: "Do we still need research on embryonic stem cells?" to which I replied a resounding "Yes." Embryonic stem cells remain the gold standard today and will remain so for the foreseeable future. If we are to maximize the pace of scientific discovery and accelerate development of new treatments for disease, we must continue to vigorously pursue all forms of stem cell research, using ES cells derived from embryos, pluripotent stem cells generated by nuclear transfer and gene-based reprogramming, and adult stem cells. Passage of the bill HR-810 originally proposed by members Castle and Degette remains a worthy goal.

In: Stem Cell Research and Science
Editor: Brenden E. Aylesworth

ISBN: 978-1-60876-083-1
© 2010 Nova Science Publishers, Inc.

Chapter 6

Testimony of John K. Fraser

John K. Fraser

Good morning, my name is John Fraser, and I am Principal Scientist at Cytori Therapeutics Inc, a publically-traded stem cell company in San Diego, California. Cytori is at the forefront of brining adult stem cells to patients, as we are currently selling a stem cell-based product in Europe, are conducting three separate clinical trials, and have a technology, which has been used in over 200 patient procedures.

From my graduate studies in New Zealand, through to a postdoctoral and then faculty appointment at UCLA, and now at Cytori, my entire research career has been centered on adult stem cells.

The topic of today's meeting is consideration of stem cells as the future of medicine. Indeed, stem cells will be an important part of the clinical armamentarium going forward. But this is nothing new; hematopoietic stem cells have been used in medicine for at least 50 years. In pioneering work started in the late 1950's E. Donnall Thomas performed bone marrow transplant studies that ultimately led to the award of the Nobel Prize for Medicine in 1990 (1-3). Many consider 1961 as the birth date of the stem cell field as that was the year that James E Till and Ernest A McCulloch published research (4) that led to the description of the first stem cell (5), the hematopoietic stem cell; which is still widely considered to be the model for all adult stem cells (6).

Hematopoietic stem cells make bone marrow transplantation possible. This is because they have the ability to regenerate the entire blood system of the recipient for the rest of that person's life. Simply put, hematopoietic stem cells are the regenerative engine of the blood system.

In my opinion, this is a key point of distinction between adult stem cells and embryonic stem cells. Embryonic stem cells are capable of immense proliferation and essentially universal plasticity. This is because they are, first and foremost, developmental cells; they are derived from a cell mass from which the entire organism develops.

By contrast, adult stem cells are, first and foremost, regenerative cells, responsible for maintaining and healing organs and tissues in the face of daily wear and tear, injury, and disease. They are, by their nature, repair cells; they activate in response to a need and shut off once healing is completed. One way to look at this is to view embryonic stem cells as responsible for generating all the tissues of an organism, while adult stem cells are responsible for maintaining and healing them.

The natural role of adult stem cells in repair and regeneration makes them ideally suited for clinical use. This has been proven in tens of thousands of bone marrow transplant patients in the last 40 years. This paradigm is now increasingly being repeated as other adult cell types associated with repair and regeneration are being applied in different diseases.

For example, Cytori has initiated several clinical studies using cells obtained from the patient's own fat tissue, which is recognized as one of the richest and most accessible sources for adult stem cells. The goal of these studies is to bring forth new treatments for the millions of patients suffering from heart disease as well as to help reconstruction breast defects in women who have undergone partial mastectomy. We also intend to start studies in intervertebral disc repair and potentially several other clinical applications, which look promising.

Other researchers have published case reports and clinical studies using fat tissue-derived stem cells in treating certain types of wound (7-9), in treating complications associated with bone marrow transplantation (10-14), and in bone defects (15). Published preclinical studies have indicated potential in treating renal damage associated with chemotherapy (16), preserving dopaminergic neurons in a Parkinson's disease model (17), treating liver damage (18), ischemic (19) and hemorrhagic (20) stroke, and in tissues as disparate as the cornea (21), the lung (22,23), and the vocal fold (24).

Published clinical studies with other types of adult stem cell have shown improvement in cardiac function (25-27), in an inherited brittle bone disease (28-30), in liver disease (31-33), and peripheral vascular disease (34) to name but a few.

However, there are still many unanswered questions and clearly additional science is needed. In certain settings, the mechanisms through which adult stem cells provide benefit are not well understood. It is also not yet clear which adult stem cell sources provide greatest clinical efficacy in which diseases. These are important questions that companies such as Cytori have neither the resources nor oftentimes the incentive to address.

For example, certain potentially beneficial cell populations fall outside of patent protections limiting the incentive of companies to invest resources in proving a technology that may then be applied without their participation. Without federal support much of this promise could be left to wither on the vine.

Cytori believes that ultimately science and the marketplace will determine which technologies will succeed. We have looked at the field of regenerative medicine, performed our own basic science, pre-clinical and now clinical research and we are very optimistic regarding the ability of our approach to harness the natural role of adult stem and regenerative cells to provide clinically and cost-effective treatments for a range of human diseases in the near future. We urge your continuing support of adult stem cell research.

Thank you.

References

[1] Hamblin, T.J. E. & Donnall Thomas, M.D. (1991). *Nobel laureate 1990. Leuk Res 15*, 71.

[2] Thomas, E. D., Lochte, H. L., Jr., Lu,W. C., & Ferrebee,J. W. (1957). Intravenous infusion of bone marrow in patients receiving radiation and chemotherapy. *N Engl J Med 257,* 491-496.

[3] Thomas, E. D., Lochte, H. L., Jr., & Ferrebee,J. W. (1959). Irradiation of the entire body and marrow transplantation: some observations and comments. *Blood 14,* 1-23.

[4] Till, J. E. & McCulloch, E. A. (1961). A direct measurement of the radiation sensitivity of normal mouse bone marrow cells. *Radiat Res 14,* 213-222.

[5] Becker, A. J., McCulloch, E., & Till,J. (1963). Cytological demonstration of the clonal nature of spleen colonies derived from transplanted mouse marrow cells. *Nature 197,* 452-454

[6]   Bryder, D., Rossi, D. J., & Weissman, I. L. (2006). Hematopoietic stem cells: the paradigmatic tissue-specific stem cell. *Am J Pathol* **169**, 338-346.

[7]   Garcia-Olmo, D., Garcia-Arranz, M., Garcia, L. G., Cuellar, E. S., Blanco, I. F., Prianes, L. A., Montes, J. A., Pinto, F. L., Marcos, D. H., & Garcia-Sancho, L. (2003). Autologous stem cell transplantation for treatment of rectovaginal fistula in perianal Crohn's disease: a new cell-based therapy. *Int J Colorectal Dis* **18**, 451-454.

[8]   Garcia-Olmo, D., Garcia-Arranz, M., Herreros, D., Pascual, I., Peiro, C., & Rodriguez-Montes, J. A. (2005). A phase I clinical trial of the treatment of Crohn's fistula by adipose mesenchymal stem cell transplantation. *Dis Colon Rectum* **48**, 1416-1423.

[9]   Alvarez, P. D., Garcia-Arranz, M., Georgiev-Hristov, T., & Garcia-Olmo, D. (2008). A new bronchoscopic treatment of tracheomediastinal fistula using autologous adipose-derived stem cells. *Thorax* **63**, 374-376.

[10] Fang, B., Song, Y., Liao, L., Zhang, Y., & Zhao, R. C. (2007). Favorable response to human adipose tissuederived mesenchymal stem cells in steroid-refractory acute graft-versus-host disease. *Transplant Proc* **39**, 3358-3362.

[11] Fang, B., Song, Y., Lin, Q., Zhang, Y., Cao, Y., Zhao, R. C., & Ma, Y. (2007). Human adipose tissue-derived mesenchymal stromal cells as salvage therapy for treatment of severe refractory acute graft-vs.-host disease in two children. *Pediatr Transplant* **11**, 814-817.

[12] Fang, B., Song, Y., Zhao, R. C., Han, Q., & Cao, Y. (2007). Treatment of resistant pure red cell aplasia after major abo-incompatible bone marrow transplantation with human adipose tissue-derived mesenchymal stem cells. *Am J Hematol* **82**, 772-773.

[13] Fang, B., Song, Y. P., Liao, L. M., Han, Q., & Zhao, R. C. (2006). Treatment of severe therapy-resistant acute graft-versus-host disease with human adipose tissue-derived mesenchymal stem cells. *Bone Marrow Transplant* **38**, 389-390.

[14] Fang, B., Song, Y., Zhao, R. C., Han, Q., & Lin, Q. (2007). Using human adipose tissue-derived mesenchymal stem cells as salvage therapy for hepatic graft-versus-host disease resembling acute hepatitis. *Transplant Proc* **39**, 1710-1713.

[15] Lendeckel, S., Jodicke, A., Christophis, P., Heidinger, K., Wolff, J., Fraser, J. K., Hedrick, M. H., Berthold, L., & Howaldt, H. P. (2004). Autologous

stem cells (adipose) and fibrin glue used to treat widespread traumatic calvarial defects: case report. *J Craniomaxillofac. Surg 32,* 370-373.

[16] Bi, B., Schmitt, R., Israilova, M., Nishio, H., & Cantley, L. G. (2007). Stromal cells protect against acute tubular injury via an endocrine effect. *J Am Soc Nephrol 18,* 2486-2496.

[17] McCoy, M. K., Martinez, T. N., Ruhn, K. A., Wrage, P. C., Keefer, E. W., Botterman, B. R., Tansey, K. E., & Tansey, M. G. (2007). Autologous transplants of Adipose-Derived Adult Stromal (ADAS) cells afford dopaminergic neuroprotection in a model of Parkinson's disease. *Exp Neurol.*

[18] Banas,A., Tokuhara,T., Teratani,T., Quinn,G., Yamamoto,Y., & Ochiya,T. Adipose tissue-derived mesenchymal stem cells as a source of human hepatocytes. *Hepatology 45,* (in press) (2007).

[19] Kang, S. K., Lee, D. H., Bae, Y. C., Kim, H. K., Baik, S. Y., & Jung, J. S. (2003). Improvement of neurological deficits by intracerebral transplantation of human adipose tissue-derived stromal cells after cerebral ischemia in rats. *Exp Neurol. 183,* 355-366.

[20] Kim, J. M., Lee, S. T., Chu, K., Jung, K. H., Song, E. C., Kim, S. J., Sinn, D. I., Kim, J. H., Park, D. K., Kang, K. M., Hyung, H. N., Park, H. K., Won, C. II., Kim, K. H., Kim, M., Kun, I. S., & Roh, J. K. (2007). Systemic transplantation of human adipose stem cells attenuated cerebral inflammation and degeneration in a hemorrhagic stroke model. *Brain Res 1183C,* 43-50.

[21] Arnalich-Montiel, F., Pastor, S., Blazquez-Martinez, A., Fernandez-Delgado, J., Nistal, M., Alio, J. L., & De Miguel, M. P. (2007). Adipose-Derived Stem Cells are a Source for Cell Therapy of The Corneal Stroma. *Stem Cells.*

[22] Shigemura, N., Okumura, M., Mizuno, S., Imanishi, Y., Nakamura, T., & Sawa, Y. (2006). Autologous transplantation of adipose tissue-derived stromal cells ameliorates pulmonary emphysema. *Am J Transplant 6,* 2592-2600.

[23] Shigemura, N., Okumura, M., Mizuno, S., Imanishi, Y., Matsuyama, A., Shiono, H., Nakamura, T., & Sawa, Y. (2006). Lung tissue engineering technique with adipose stromal cells improves surgical outcome for pulmonary emphysema. *Am J Respir. Crit Care Med 174,* 1199-1205.

[24] Lee, B. J., Wang, S. G., Lee, J. C., Jung, J. S., Bae, Y. C., Jeong, H. J., Kim, H. W., & Lorenz, R. R. (2006). The prevention of vocal fold scarring using

autologous adipose tissue-derived stromal cells. *Cells Tissues Organs 184*, 198-204.

[25] Schachinger, V., Assmus, B., Britten, M. B., Honold, J., Lehmann, R., Teupe, C., Abolmaali, N. D., Vogl, T. J., Hofmann, W. K., Martin, H., Dimmeler, S., & Zeiher, A. M. (2004). Transplantation of progenitor cells and regeneration enhancement in acute myocardial infarction: final one-year results of the TOPCARE-AMI Trial. *J Am Coll Cardiol 44*, 1690-1699.

[26] Dimmeler, S., Burchfield, J., & Zeiher, A. M. (2008). Cell-based therapy of myocardial infarction. *Arterioscler Thromb Vasc Biol 28*, 208-216.

[27] Schachinger, V., Erbs, S., Elsasser, A., Haberbosch, W., Hambrecht, R., Holschermann, H., Yu, J., Corti, R., Mathey, D. G., Hamm, C. W., Suselbeck, T., Werner, N., Haase, J., Neuzner, J., Germing, A., Mark, B., ·Assmus, B., Tonn, T., Dimmeler, S., & Zeiher, A. M. (2006). Improved clinical outcome after intracoronary administration of bone-marrow-derived progenitor cells in acute myocardial infarction: final 1-year results of the REPAIR-AMI trial. *Eur Heart J 27*, 2775-2783.

[28] Horwitz, E. M., Gordon, P. L., Koo, W. K., Marx, J. C., Neel, M. D., McNall, R. Y., Muul, L., & Hofmann, T. (2002). Isolated allogeneic bone marrow-derived mesenchymal cells engraft and stimulate growth in children with osteogenesis imperfecta: Implications for cell therapy of bone. *Proc Natl Acad Sci U S A 99*, 8932-8937.

[29] Horwitz, E. M. (2001). Marrow mesenchymal cell transplantation for genetic disorders of bone. *Cytotherapy. 3*, 399-401.

[30] Horwitz, E. M., Prockop, D. J., Fitzpatrick, L. A., Koo, W. W., Gordon, P. L., Neel, M., Sussman, M., Orchard, P., Marx, J. C., Pyeritz, R. E., & Brenner, M. K. (1999). Transplantability and therapeutic effects of bone marrow-derived mesenchymal cells in children with osteogenesis imperfecta. *Nat Med 5*, 309-13.

[31] Sakaida, I. (2008). Autologous bone marrow cell infusion therapy for liver cirrhosis. *J Gastroenterol Hepatol*.

[32] Sakaida, I. (2006). Clinical application of bone marrow cell transplantation for liver diseases. *J Gastroenterol 41*, 93-94.

[33] Sakaida, I., Terai, S., & Okita, K. (2005). Use of bone marrow cells for the development of cellular therapy in liver diseases. *Hepatol Res 31*, 195-196.

[34] Kajiguchi, M., Kondo, T., Izawa, H., Kobayashi, M., Yamamoto, K., Shintani, S., Numaguchi, Y., Naoe, T., Takamatsu, J., Komori, K., &

Murohara, T. (2007). Safety and efficacy of autologous progenitor cell transplantation for therapeutic angiogenesis in patients with critical limb ischemia. *Circ J 71*, 196-201.

NIH Research Contract and Grant Funding Received by Dr Fraser

1R44HL076045 "Adipose Derived Cell Therapy for Myocardial Infarction" awarded by the National Heart, Lung, and Blood Institute of the National Institutes of Health. January 2004 to July 2006: Total $950,000

1R43HL088871-01 "Adipose Tissue-Derived Cells for Vascular Cell Therapy" awarded by the National Heart, Lung, and Blood Institute of the National Institutes of Health. September 2007 to August 2008: Total $250,000

1N01HB067142 "Collection and Storage Centers for Clinical Research on Umbilical Cord Blood Stem and Progenitor Cell Transplantation". September 1996 – September 2001: Total ~$11 million.

In: Stem Cell Research and Science
Editor: Brenden E. Aylesworth

ISBN: 978-1-60876-083-1
© 2010 Nova Science Publishers, Inc.

Chapter 7

Testimony on Stem Cell Science: The Foundation for Future Cures before the U.S. House of Representatives Subcommittee on Health of the Committee on Energy and Commerce

John Gearhart and C. Michael Armstron

Mr. Chairman and Members of the Subcommittee, I am John Gearhart, a stem cell biologist at Johns Hopkins Medicine. I am pleased to appear before you to discuss the foundation for future cures through stem cell science.

It is rare that a field of scientific research can have both an enormous potential impact of human health and quality of life and be a fount of new basic research discovery. What crystallized the scientific and medical communities' interest in stem cell research was the derivation of human embryonic stem cell lines. These cell lines are unique in that they are capable of forming all the different cell types (>220) that are present in the body (a property that is referred to as pluripotentiality) and they can produce more cells like themselves indefinitely (self-renew). This development, first reported ten years ago, has been among the most heralded as well as contentious issues of the modern scientific era. Heralded, as now we had in the laboratory a source of cells from which we could grow any and all cells of the human body for much needed replacement therapies and contentious, because embryos are destroyed to derive the cells. No wonder that stem cell research has impacted many areas of our society – science, medicine, religion, ethics, policy and economics. Seldom has a week gone by without some new revelation about stem cells reaching the front pages of the press or the top news stories of the day and what this means for our society, invariably hyped. It is recognized that stem cell research has the potential to revolutionize the practice of medicine and to improve the quality of life and in some cases, the length of life for many people suffering from devastating illnesses and injuries. Also, it is believed by many that there will be no realm of medicine that will not be impacted by stem cell research.

Research over the past ten years is setting the foundation for the use of embryonic stem cells and the knowledge derived from this research for developing and designing therapies, therapies that will be safe as well as effective. To envision what lies ahead for the use of these cells in human therapies, it is informative to mention the progress that has been made over the past decade while keeping in mind that the progress made by US investigators has been compromised by current policy on federal funding. In the very first Congressional hearing on these stem cells (December 2, 1998, Before the Senate Appropriations Committee, Subcommittee on Labor, Health and Human Services, Education and Related Agencies) and one in which I had participated, Harold Varmus, MD, then the Director of the National Institutes of Health (now the President of the Memorial Sloan-Kettering Cancer Center) outlined the potential uses of these cells in biomedicine and it is appropriate to use his list in evaluating what has transpired in laboratories since then.

(Varmus) At the most fundamental level, pluripotent stem cells could help us to understand the complex events that occur during human development. A primary goal of this work would be the most basic kind of research --the identification of the factors involved in the cellular decision-making process that determines cell specialization. We know that turning genes on and off is central to this process, but we do not know much about these "decision-making" genes or what turns them on or off. Some of our most serious diseases, like cancer, are due to abnormal cell differentiation and growth. A deeper understanding of normal cell processes will allow us to further delineate the fundamental errors that cause these deadly illnesses.

There is no question that we have learned a great deal about these stem cells and the molecular mechanisms underlying the bases of pluripotentiality and of cell differentiation, that is, the conversion of these cells into one of the types of specialized cells of the body. This is what we call basic science, a prerequisite first step in understanding cellular processes. We have utilized studies of other organisms to first give us insight into these mechanisms and then confirmed these mechanisms or variations on these mechanisms in the human cells. Much of our progress has been informed by such studies and as has been pointed out recently by Bruce Alberts, Ph.D., there are no shortcuts to medical progress: *But, as has been repeatedly demonstrated, the shortest path to medical breakthroughs may not come from a direct attack against a specific disease. Critical medical insights frequently arise from attempts to understand fundamental mechanisms in organisms that are much easier to study than humans; in particular, from studies of bacteria, yeasts, insects, plants, and worms. For this reason, an overemphasis on "translational" biomedical research (which focuses on a particular disease) would be counterproductive, even for those who care only about disease prevention and cures. (Bruce Alberts, Shortcuts to Medical Progress? Science Vol 319, 28 March 2008).* Embryonic stem cells provide another link in the biomedical investigation and discovery chain that leads to human application.

So, we now know a handful of the critical genes and of the regulation of the expression of these genes that enable cells to be pluripotential. This knowledge was at the basis of the most recent and exciting development in our field in which skin cells were converted to cells that had properties of embryonic stem cells by the addition of just a few genes to the cells. The skin cells had these genes but they were not being expressed. Adding exogenous version genes that were expressed caused these cells to be reprogrammed, eventually expressing their own, endogenous genes. The embryonic stem cell-like cells are called induced pluripotent stem (iPS) cells. This is a major paradigm shift in stem cell biology and I will comment more on this later but it was through the study of embryonic stem cells that this advance was made.

There have now been hundreds of research reports on studies of in which embryonic stem cells are differentiating to specialized cells. We are learning the mechanisms involved in the earliest decisions made by cells to become neurons or gut cells or muscle cells, etc. It has been know for decades that cell-cell interactions in the embryo determine the fates of cells during development as summarized by the Noble laureate Hans Spemann (1943): *We are standing and walking with parts of our body which we could have used for thinking if they had been developed in another position in the embryo.* With these embryonic stem cells in culture, we are learning how different factors influence cell fate decisions. By experimentally manipulating these factors we can then direct cell differentiation to a desired cell type through the use of growth factors, attempting to mimic the environment of the embryo.

Personally, I have been interested in human embryology and development for decades and have felt strongly as Samuel Taylor Coleridge (1934) stated so beautifully: *The history of man for the nine months preceding his birth would probably be far more interesting and contain events of far greater moment, than all the three-score and ten years that follow.* These stem cells have provided a unique resource to learn about the biologic mechanisms underlying our development, both normal and abnormal, so that we may eventually understand the basis of birth defects and perhaps guide us in correcting these malformations, etc. We have learned much about the mechanisms of cell decision making in the early embryo, such as within the conceptus, becoming embryonic or extra-embryonic, and within the germ layers of the embryo, what determines cell fate. In our own current work with embryonic stem cells, we have recently discovered ~40 new genes that are critical to the formation of the heart and great vessels. There are many other examples for the use of these important cells in studying human development.

Recent findings have discovered and solidified the understanding that many of the same cellular mechanisms found in the development of a tissue or organ play critical roles when rebuilding or regenerating that tissue. Investigators have gone on to show that manipulation of these developmental factors, the understanding for which has been often discovered, expanded and/or validated in embryonic stem cells, can greatly influence regenerative capacity, even recovering the capacity to regenerate in animals that did not possess it. It is of the outmost importance that studies continue in order to discover these and utilize this knowledge in designing therapies for the many maladies affecting us. As all of you have observed, we humans don't regenerated body parts like some of our lower relatives in the animal kingdom. Imagine the possibility of harnessing the capacity of zebrafish, for example, who using the same families of genes that we use in the development of our heart can regrow a large part of their heart when amputated. We must determine the reasons why humans fail to display this capacity in most organs, emboldened by the knowledge that our livers can regenerate, in order to combat many common debilitating diseases such as heart attacks and strokes.

(Varmus) Human pluripotent stem cell research could also dramatically change the way we develop drugs and test them for safety and efficacy. Rather than evaluating safety and efficacy of a candidate drug in an animal model of a human disease, these drugs could be tested against a human cell line that had

been developed to mimic the disease processes. This would not replace whole animal and human testing, but it would streamline the road to discovery. Only the most effective and safest candidate would be likely to graduate to whole animal and then human testing.

There have now been many examples of use of what are called high throughput screens for testing the effect of various chemicals, molecules and drugs on the stem cells and their specialized derivatives. The use of this approach for studies with 'diseased' cells is just beginning as embryonic stem cells have been derived from embryos diagnosed with mutations that can lead to disease later in life.

(Varmus) Perhaps the most far-reaching potential application of human pluripotent stem cells is the generation of cells and tissue that could be used for transplantation, so-called cell therapies. Many diseases and disorders result from disruption of cellular function or destruction of tissues of the body. Today, donated organs and tissues are often used to replace the function of ailing or destroyed tissue. Unfortunately, the number of people suffering from these disorders far outstrips the number of organs available for transplantation. Pluripotent stem cells stimulated to develop into specialized cells offer the possibility of a renewable source of replacement cells and tissue to treat a myriad of diseases, conditions and disabilities including Parkinson's and Alzheimer's disease, spinal cord injury, stroke, burns, heart disease, diabetes, osteoarthritis and rheumatoid arthritis. There is almost no realm of medicine that might not be touched by this innovation

There are now many reports on the use of embryonic stem cell sources of cells for grafting into animals with various injuries or that serve as models for a variety of human diseases. The results have been highly variable (as it has been using stem cells from any source, adult or embryonic) but in many cases, they are encouraging. Our laboratory has been working with cell-based therapies for the heart. Currently there are no adult stem cells that have been identified to date that have shown robust cardiac muscle formation in vivo (in the heart), or for that matter, in vitro (in the dish). We and other laboratories have identified a stem cell that gives rise to most of the cells within the heart and these cells, when grafted to infarcted rodent hearts robustly undergo cardiac muscle formation, integrate into the heart and restore function.

There are three further important points that I want to make in considering the future of providing cures or ameliorating diseases and injuries through stem cell science.

Time frame for developing safe and effective therapies.

Where disease is involved, we must determine the underlying pathogenesis of the disease and stop it. I have talked only about having a source of cells (or the knowledge of how to control cell fates) in establishing a foundation for future therapies. What is as important, is the understanding of the pathogenesis of devastating diseases for we must stop this process for grafted cells will surely succumb to the same fate.

How do the iPS cells factor into the future?

Quite simply I believe that they are important part of the future. They require further vetting as true embryonic stem cells. At the moment, we can only measure what can measure with embryonic stem cells and induced pluripotent stem cells. More must be learned about each. They represent a powerful example of our goal to instruct our cells to do what we want; but this is just the beginning. Is this a farewell to embryonic stem cells in research? Not at all, for they represent the gold standard. For my studies focused on human embryology, I will continue to use embryonic cells but, like many of my colleagues, I will vigorously pursue the direct reprogramming of adult cells.

Summary

Mr. Chairman, I am grateful to you for providing a forum to discuss this promising arena of science and medicine. Learning to instruct our cells to get them to do what we want is the ultimate control of our own cells and the basis of future medicine. Based on current research results with stem cells, the future is, as Yogi Berra has said, not what it used to be. We look to stem cells not only to provide cells for replacements in therapies, but also to provide us with the knowledge of how cells work and to use this information to instruct patients' cells to effect repair and regeneration of damaged or diseased tissues. We must recognize that the development therapies that are safe and effective is going to take time and resources and that circumspection is not a retreat from promise. I would be pleased to answer any questions you might have.

In: Stem Cell Research and Science
Editor: Brenden E. Aylesworth

ISBN: 978-1-60876-083-1
© 2010 Nova Science Publishers, Inc.

Chapter 8

Written Testimony of Weyman Johnson, Individual Living with Multiple Sclerosis, Chairman of the Board, National Multiple Sclerosis Society, Energy and Commerce Committee Subcommittee on Health U.S. House of Representatives

Weyman Johnson

Summary of my personal and family experiences with a chronic, disabling disease.

Speak to a patient perspective on my own diagnosis with multiple sclerosis.

Speak to the position of a national voluntary health organization, as chairman of the board of the National Multiple Sclerosis Society.

Speak to the need for continued research and the hope it brings for people living with chronic diseases and conditions nationwide.

Support the need for the Committee and Congress to remain committed to legislation like the Stem Cell Research Enhancement Act.

Embryonic stem cell research holds an incredibly unique promise for people living with chronic diseases and conditions, and the progress made to date on embryonic stem cell lines should not be abandoned.

Thank you Chairman Pallone and Ranking Member Deal. Thank you members of the Committee. I am honored to be invited to speak here today among many distinguished panelists and to represent patients who live with chronic disease.

Many diseases could benefit from expanded embryonic stem cell research. But today I will focus on one—multiple sclerosis. Not because it is more important than others, but because I know multiple sclerosis.

I remember multiple sclerosis and how it entered my life as a child, in 1964, just barely 13 years old. My father received a diagnosis of MS suddenly. He died in 2001. His sister, my aunt Allene, also had MS. Research into this disease, into genetics was just starting to evolve in the 1960s.

There were good doctors then, but they did not recognize a genetic connection. They said MS in my family was a mere coincidence. Because of research, we now know that is not true.

My own sister, who's only a few years older than I, lives with MS. She uses a power wheelchair, her hands don't work well anymore, she can no longer teach the way she did, or play the piano the way she did. A few years after she was diagnosed, so was I. We hate this disease, its impact on our family, and the threat it poses to our future generations.

We are making progress into the genetic factors involved in multiple sclerosis. However there are still more questions than answers. The research must continue.

I remember being told that MS is a disease that doesn't affect my friends in the African American community. This is only for white people from Minnesota. With good science, we have found that's not true. The research must continue.

We also used to hear that this disease does not happen to children. But that is not true either. We now know there are thousands of children in the United States, thousands of children throughout the world, who live with this disease. The research must continue.

Before 1993, there were no treatments at all for multiple sclerosis. Now we have six. But there is a wide spectrum among people living with MS. Most of the therapies will only work for those of us on the lucky end of the spectrum like me. But for people like my sister, on the more unlucky end, there's still not much out there that provides effective treatment. So the research must continue.

Every hour, someone new is diagnosed with MS. It's an unpredictable, often disabling disease of the central nervous system. The progress, severity, and specific symptoms of MS in any one person still cannot be predicted. The cause is unknown, and there is no cure. But embryonic stem cell research holds an incredibly unique promise to repair nerve cells, to slow the progression of MS, to help find a cure.

One area that holds great promise, but is often misunderstood, is Somatic Cell Nuclear Transfer. We have seen some exciting breakthroughs. But as with all science, this research takes time. We are still exploring this avenue for medical research. I have hope that SCNT will succeed because of its promise to repair nerve cells, creating new tissues, and more. I know that researchers are focused on the idea of creating cells and tissues for transplantation and research. They are trying to understand how different genes are turned on and off. They are not focused on cloning. I know that as we explore somatic cell nuclear transfer research more, we will see greater potential for developing individualized cell and tissue therapies. That holds great promise for people living with MS like me, whose body's own defense system is attacking the myelin surrounding and protecting our central nervous system.

I am but one person living with a chronic disease. But I am also fortunate to serve as chairman of the board of the National Multiple Sclerosis Society. We believe that all promising avenues of research that could lead to new ways to prevent, repair, slow the progression, or cure MS *must* be explored, with adherence to the strictest ethical and procedural guidelines. The National Multiple Sclerosis Society believes that all promising avenues of research that could lead to the cure or prevention of multiple sclerosis or relieve its symptoms must be explored. The Society supports the Stem Cell Research Enhancement Act to expand the number of approved stem cell lines that are available for federally funded research. The Society supports the conduct of scientifically meritorious medical research, including research using human cells, in accordance with federal, state, and local laws and with adherence to the strictest ethical and procedural guidelines.

Research on all types of stem cells is critical because we have no way of knowing which type of stem cell will be of the most value in MS research. Stem cells — adult or embryonic — could have the potential to be used to protect and rebuild tissues that are damaged by MS, and to deliver molecules that foster repair or protect vulnerable tissues from further injury.

So I ask you to expand the federal policy on embryonic stem cell research and ensure that research continues ... for the more than 400,000 other Americans who live with MS and 100 million Americans with other diseases and conditions. Research on all types of stem cells is critical because we have no way of knowing at this point which type of stem cell will be of the most value ... for multiple sclerosis, for Parkinson's, for Alzheimer's, for cancer, for heart disease, for spinal cord and brain injuries, for many other conditions.

Just like with genetics and race and age, there is so much left to learn about how to treat and cure MS ... about how to treat and cure other diseases. Expanding our embryonic stem cell research is just one avenue. But it is an avenue of research that must continue. Federal barriers must be lifted.

You might see that I am not the only person living with MS on Capitol Hill today. *Hundreds* of MS activists are visiting with their legislators on the Hill right now, talking about the need to advance medical research.

Embryonic stem cell research remains one of the most promising avenues of research to cure diseases and end suffering. I am not a scientist, but I am an observer of science. And I know that science is a matter that requires some patience. That's why we must expand the important work done to date with embryonic stem cell lines. The research must continue. So we can improve the lives of people with chronic diseases and conditions. So we can improve the lives of families for generations to come. For my grandchildren and for yours.

We need your commitment to not give up on legislation like the Stem Cell Research Enhancement Act. We don't have the luxury of time. Like many others who live with a chronic disease, I know ... maybe not today, maybe not next week, but I pray soon ... with patience and continued research ... that there will be no more disease. Thank you for helping us move closer, and thank you for your time.

National Multiple Sclerosis Society Policy Position Embryonic Stem Cell Lines Available for Federally Funded Research

Position

The National Multiple Sclerosis Society believes that all promising avenues of research that could lead to the cure or prevention of multiple sclerosis or relieve its symptoms must be explored. The Society supports the Stem Cell

Research Enhancement Act (H.R. 3 and S. 5) to expand the number of approved stem cell lines that are available for federally funded research.

The Society supports the conduct of scientifically meritorious medical research, including research using human cells, in accordance with federal, state, and local laws and with adherence to the strictest ethical and procedural guidelines. Research on all types of stem cells is critical because we have no way of knowing which type of stem cell will be of the most value in MS research. Stem cells — adult or embryonic — could have the potential to be used to protect and rebuild tissues that are damaged by MS, and to deliver molecules that foster repair or protect vulnerable tissues from further injury.

Request

We urge Congress to support the Stem Cell Research Enhancement Act of 2007 (H.R. 3 and S. 5) at all levels of the legislative process. This legislation would increase the number of approved embryonic stem cell lines that can be used in federally funded research by allowing new lines to be generated from embryos that have been donated for research purposes by people using the services of in vitro fertilization clinics, while establishing important ethical protections.

Supporting Rationale

There is broad agreement that the policy limiting the number of stem cell lines available for federally funded research is flawed.

An insufficient supply of stem cell lines currently exists, as only 22 of the 70 approved lines are available to researchers. In addition, all of the available lines are contaminated by nutrients from mouse feeder cells. Many in the scientific community believe that these stem cell lines are unsuitable for research and hinder U.S. scientists' ability to capitalize on the potential breakthroughs from embryonic stem cell research.

At the same time, it has become increasingly clear that stem cell research holds tremendous promise for MS and many other diseases and disorders. Research suggests that stem cells might have many uses: for delivery of growth factors and drugs, for tissue culture systems for drug and gene discovery, for understanding and modeling MS, and for repairing or protecting brain tissue.

However, our scientific advisors have told us that we still don't know which type of stem cells will be most valuable for MS research, and thus we must support policies that promote the conduct of research using all types of stem cells.

In: Stem Cell Research and Science
Editor: Brenden E. Aylesworth

ISBN: 978-1-60876-083-1
© 2010 Nova Science Publishers, Inc.

Chapter 9

Testimony for "Stem Cell Science: The Foundation for Future Cures" before the Subcommittee on Health of the Committee on Energy and Commerce

Amit N Patel

Chairman and members of the Committee, thank you for inviting me to testify before you. My name is Amit Patel. Please note that the testimony I am giving today is my own opinion and not necessarily that of the institution where I am currently employed. I am a translational scientist for cardiovascular diseases where my research is focused on working with regenerative therapies taking the science from the lab bench to the patients. I am also a cardiovascular surgeon who on daily basis sees patients who have exhausted all medical and surgical options available who may benefit from the science of stem cell research.

My goal today is to give both a scientific and real life perspective of the impact that cardiovascular disease has in the United States and potential use of stem cell therapies.

Cardiovascular Disease

Heart disease is the leading cause of death in the United States. Nearly 930,000 Americans die of cardiovascular diseases each year, which amounts to one death every 33 seconds. About 70 million Americans have some form of cardiovascular disease, which is responsible for more than 6 million hospitalizations each year. There are over a one million patients with heart attacks every year, along with six million patients with chronic angina (chest pain), and five millions patients with heart failure. In 2005, the cost of heart disease and stroke in the United States exceeded $394 billion: $242 billion for health care expenditures and $152 billion for lost productivity from death and disability. Patients with end-stage cardiovascular disease have over $30 billion dollars in health care expenditures per year. Also, up to 20% of patients over the age 70 have limb ischemia.

Problem

The patients with end stage cardiovascular disease have at least one of two major problems:

Heart failure, where there is inadequate pumping function of heart due to decreased blood supply or lack of sufficient muscle.
Critical limb ischemia, where there is inadequate blood supply to the leg.

Current Treatment Options

Heart failure management involves optimal treatment with oral and/or intravenous medications along with surgical therapies. As patients continue to deteriorate the use of artificial hearts and heart transplantation remain the gold standard for end-stage therapy. There are many problems with the surgical options such as infection, stroke, rejection, and the overall costs associated with treatment. However, even with all these options there are limited organs for transplant and fifty percent of endstage heart failure patients die within five years.
Critical limb ischemia management involves oral medical therapy followed by surgical revascularization by bypass grafts. If the graft fails and further

reoperative therapy is not possible, then amputation of the leg is performed. This problem is more severe in patients who also have diabetes.

The Role of Stem Cells

Based on the current science, human stem cells have been shown both in a lab dish and in the pre-human work to make new blood vessels and in rare cases new heart muscle.

Current Clinical Therapies

Human stem cell therapies for cardiovascular disease have been performed under legitimate clinical trials since early 2000. The first group of patients had cells from thigh muscle (skeletal myoblasts) injected into their heart at the time of coronary bypass surgery hoping to grow new heart muscle in Europe. The early data demonstrated some issues with the therapy but larger trials were performed which also did not show significant improvement in heart function. This was truly an example of too rapid translation which could have destroyed the field. However, when these cells where used in a heart failure population and delivered via a catheter in U.S., the results where positive and have led to a large scale clinical trial. Also, using bone marrow cell therapy for the same patient population, both surgically and catheter based delivery has been performed in over one thousand patients in registered trials demonstrating no safety issues. This is the most important issue when performing translational therapies even though all the mechanisms of action have not been defined. As patient safety has been established, the next goal is to identify the patient population which may benefit the most from this therapy, which in the lab dish and pre-human work has shown to grow blood vessels and may improve cardiac muscle function. In these early clinical trials there has been modest improvement in heart function but there has been a significant decrease in adverse events, readmission for heart failure and new heart attacks in the randomized controlled studies. It is true that improvement in overall pumping has not been as large as most people had anticipated but that is most likely related to baseline function of the patient being enrolled in the studies. The analysis of the more severely impaired patients has shown a very dramatic increase which could not be attributed to medical therapy alone. The problem is, that most of these trials have been conducted in Europe or South America.

Similarly, the use of bone marrow stem cells for critical limb ischemia has also been studied since 2000. Most of the early clinical work was performed in Japan, with later translation to Europe and then most recently to the U.S. There has been a decrease in the rate of amputations which has been significant enough that the German government has approved certain centers of expertise which perform the therapy on patients as standard of care and obtain reimbursement from the equivalent of CMS.

Both of these examples are of the first generation of cardiovascular cell therapy. There are many other multi- and pluri-potent stem cells which also have potential for clinical use in cardiovascular disease but the safety still needs to be established before large scale clinical trials are performed such as adipose (fat), amniotic, menstrual, umbilical cord, cardiac stem ,cells, fetal, and embryonic. Some of these cells are in phase I safety trials both here in the U.S. and Europe. I have attached a table below which shows some of the larger cardiovascular studies in the U.S. and the rest of the world based on the international registry clinicaltrials.gov.

Phase III	Country	# Patients	Funding	Results
Acute Myocardial Infarction	Germany	200, 800 pending	Government/ Private/ Corporate	Safe, Mild improvement in heart function and decease mid term adverse events
Acute Myocardial Infarction	Brazil	300	Government	Ongoing
Heart Failure	Brazil	300	Government	Ongoing
Limb Ischemia	Germany	90	Government	Ongoing
Phase II/III				
Heart Failure- myoblasts	USA	390	Corporate	Ongoing
CABG + cells	Germany	100	Government	Pending
Phase II				
Chronic Angina	USA	120	Corporate	Completed awaiting results

Problems in Clinical Use

There are a number of clinical issues related to translation into reliable therapy. I have listed them below but also have attached a supplement which goes into further detail for each question: 1. What is the best source of stem cells? 2. Is a variety or combination of cells required for different types of heart disease? 3. What are the doses of cells required in humans compared to animals? 4. Are therapeutic doses available? 5. If so, what will be necessary to acquire them? 6. What is the best delivery method for the cells into the heart? 7. When is the best time after myocardial injury to deliver the cells? 8. Are the cells going to stay in the heart and, if not, where do they go and will they cause any harm? 9. How do we follow applied cells over time? 10. Will a tissue engineered scaffold be required to enhance effect? 11. Is it worth the risk to the patient?

Roles of the National Institutes of Health & Food and Drug Administration

The NIH has done a great job in terms of supporting cardiovascular cell based therapies by developing Cell Therapy Network, Heart Failure Network, and the Cardiac Surgery Network. They will all play a significant role in answering the above questions and advancing clinical cardiac cell therapy and the science that is needed to make it a reliable, safe and reproducible therapy.

The FDA has also been very helpful in approving clinical trials with adult based cell therapies. However, the use of both outside basic and clinical scientists in the field early in the development and approval of the trials may expedite approval but more importantly help in ensuring safety to the patients, which is most important.

Summary

Cardiovascular cell therapies using the first generation adult stem cell have great potential to help our patients today. The science needs to continue to improve and help support the safety and efficacy of the therapies. Continued development of other multipotent stem cells along with tissue engineering to make new large blood vessels, heart valves, and the entire heart are the future of cardiac cell therapy. However, significant improvement in the amount of funding is required to keep pace with other countries but most importantly help our patients here in the U.S. I am a realist that these early therapies are a treatment for cardiovascular disease and not a cure. They are experimental but without our current work, the future cures that everyone hopes for and needs will be very difficult if not impossible to achieve.

In: Stem Cell Research and Science
Editor: Brenden E. Aylesworth

ISBN: 978-1-60876-083-1
© 2010 Nova Science Publishers, Inc.

Chapter 10

Adult Stem Cell Recipient for the Heart

Douglas T. Rice

My name is Douglas T. Rice. I am 62 years old, have Congestive Heart Disease, and Diabetes. I could be one of over 750,000 people that die in the United States yearly, BUT I am not dead. Not because I shouldn't be, but because there is a resolution to this problem. I am not a miracle, a phenomenon, but a living person that by the grace of God was saved from a disease that kills approximately 2,000 people daily. However, I had to travel to Bangkok, Thailand and go in debt to do something that should be readily available in the United States. I used my own Adult Stem Cells, and a simple angioplasty procedure to have my life given back to me. Your own Adult Stem Cells have so much more to give than we give them credit for; a lot of other diseases are being treated successfully by just using the Adult Stem Cells.

My story is simple. In 1992 I had my first Heart Attack and was also diagnosed with Diabetes. That same year my mother died of Congestive Heart Failure and Diabetes, just like what I have. Also, just last year my sister died of what I have. I have had numerous Heart Attacks and Diabetes episodes as well as having to be jump-started at least three times. I have had a TMR (Trans Myocardial Revascularization), a procedure that uses a laser to drill holes in the Left Ventricle to get better blood flow--this did not help. In 1998, I was given only two years to live unless I received a Heart Transplant. Because of my

Diabetes, I did not qualify for it. We tried different things that helped and then in November of 2005, I could not walk but a few feet, had to sleep sitting up, and was just worn out. My Ejection Fraction (the amount of blood my heart pumps out each beat) was around 11% (average is 50%+) and my Cardiologist, Dr. Donald Canaday, said at best I had 4 months without a mechanical heart pump to survive. It was battery operated and I decided I did not want to be battery powered.

That night my best friend, Sheba Rice, went on the Internet looking for new heart treatments. She found TheraVitae, a company in Bangkok, Thailand, that had been having success using the Adult Stem Cells. We contacted them, went to Bangkok in January of 2006, and other than drawing blood, shipping it to Israel, and then having the Adult Stem Cells shipped back and implanted in me via a simple angioplasty procedure, it was simple. The hardest part was the 20-hour flight there. When I returned to Spokane, within a month my Ejection Fraction was tested. It was 28% and going up. I felt better than I had felt in years. I was motivated to tell the world and that is when I found out that over 750,000 Americans die every year from Heart Disease.

These 750,000 heart patients that will die do not make the mainstream press, no newspaper articles of any significance, and certainly most politicians in Washington, D.C. don't even like to discuss it. Sadly, it is a fact, if a family dies in a car wreck, children are gunned down in a school, or a disgruntled person shoots or maims his or her co-workers, it is BIG NEWS.

BUT, 750,000 people die at a rate of over 2,000 a day and no one takes the time to talk for them. Not all are old, some very young and with families and friends to care about. Most people just don't realize that they die although almost everyone knows someone that has died or will die from this disease.

The Federal Government has spent millions of dollars on Embryonic Stem Cells, but not one person has been treated and the animals tested often get tumors.

By some estimates over 400,000 people with various cancers and other diseases have been successfully treated and most are alive to talk about the Adult Stem Cell treatment using their own stem cells or ones from cord blood stem cells.

The honest experts say maybe in 10 or 20 years embryonic stem cells might have potential to treat someone, but not now, and there is something that works "NOW," the Adult Stem Cells!! What does it take to make people realize that a bird in the hand is worth two in the bush, especially when it comes to people's lives?

If you ask most people about stem cells, they only know about Embryonic, because that is all they hear about. Education, Education, Education and the Facts regarding Adult Stem Cells are the only way to succeed in moving this issue to the forefront for funding and actual treatments "NOW."

I get many calls on a daily basis because I have been treated with my Adult Stem Cells, and the most frequent question is, "Why did you have to go to Thailand?" Answer: Because there were no adult stem cell clinical trials in the US that I could participate in, and FDA has been slow to approve treatments that are being conducted overseas in countries like Thailand and Germany. My insurance did not cover the cost of this treatment (though I heard that in Germany insurance covers stem cell treatments for heart disease). I also know that much of the stem cell debate in recent years has led to drastically increased funding for embryonic stem cell research despite the fact they have not treated patients for any disease. More money needs to be spent in the United States to prevent a brain drain here for treatments, and siphoning off federal funding for embryonic stem cell research has not helped patients like me. Patients are being increasingly treated with adult stem cells, but we need drastically more federal funding for adult stem cell treatments. These cells aren't patentable, so private investment is far behind. The government should spend more on clinical trials so Americans like me can have the same chance at a treatment that I had.

Listen, I am but one man, a very lucky man to have had my best friend, Sheba Rice, find the solution on the Internet while looking for new technology for heart disease. Without her efforts, I would be in an urn on the fireplace. But, she cared and wanted me alive for whatever reason. We all need to do the same for someone we know or people that need the help. We that care need to educate everyone we meet. Not because I say it, because of the 750,000 people that will die this year!

I would get down on my knees and beg if I thought that I alone could do it. I can't. I doubt if I make a difference, but you can. You Congressmen, your Doctors, News Media and friends can make a difference. I will do whatever I can do to move this forward, but I need your help! Ask me for anything that will help and I will do my best. I am asking everyone that reads this to do their best. One day you may be where I have been, or your mother, father, brother or sister as well as relatives and friends. This is so serious I can't imagine everyone not getting involved.

Feel free to contact me if I can be of help. dtrice@douglastrice.org

Sincerely,

Douglas T. Rice

Links for information: www.vescell.com

In: Stem Cell Research and Science
Editor: Brenden E. Aylesworth

ISBN: 978-1-60876-083-1
© 2010 Nova Science Publishers, Inc.

Chapter 11

Stem Cell Science: The Foundation of Future Cures

Elias A. Zerhouni

Good morning, Mr. Chairman, Ranking Member Deal and Members of the Subcommittee. I am Elias Zerhouni, the Director of the National Institutes of Health (NIH), an agency of the U.S. Department of Health and Human Services (HHS), and I am pleased to appear before you today to testify about the science of stem cell research. I look forward to discussing ongoing federal support of both embryonic and non-embryonic stem cell research and scientific progress, including the recently published findings on induced pluripotent stem cells and other updates provided during the NIH Symposium on Cell-Based Therapies, which we hosted just two days ago.

Stem cell research has the potential to lead to therapies for injuries and illnesses that could not even have been imagined when I first began studying medicine. As this new field of discovery advances, nothing we have learned has dissuaded us from the belief that these cells, representing the building blocks of life itself, offer the possibility of becoming a renewable source of replacement cells and tissues to treat such common diseases and disorders as Parkinson's disease, spinal cord injury, stroke, burns, heart disease, diabetes, osteoarthritis, and rheumatoid arthritis.

A great deal of progress has already occurred. When I first became the Director of NIH, scientists were still struggling with learning how to grow embryonic stem cell lines. Since then, experiments have occurred in animals where embryonic stem cells actually replaced damaged cells and tissues. But we have a very long way to go.

The Need for Research to Explore the Potential of Human Stem Cells

Stem cells can multiply without changing – that is, self-renew – or can differentiate to produce specialized cell types. This ability to renew and eventually replace damaged cells and tissues fuels the excitement of stem cell researchers across the world. But all stem cells do not come from the same source; they have different characteristics and are difficult to harness and grow. Stem cells have been derived from both embryonic and non-embryonic tissues, and these cell types have different properties. Both pluripotent and nonpluripotent types show potential for developing treatments for human diseases and injuries, and there are many ways in which they might be used in basic and clinical research. We are still early in the learning process. This is an exciting but new field of discovery, and additional research is needed to realize the potential of stem cells and their uses. Before we reach the promised land of stem cell therapies, scientists must learn to reliably manipulate the cells so that they possess the necessary characteristics for successful differentiation, transplantation, and engraftment.

To be useful for transplant purposes, differentiated stem cells must:

Proliferate extensively and generate sufficient quantities of specialized cells;
Differentiate into the desired cell type(s);
Survive in the recipient after transplant;
Integrate into the surrounding tissue after transplant;
Function appropriately for extended periods of time; and
Avoid harming the recipient.

As this field of research advances, stem cells will yield still unknown information about the complex events that occur during the initial stages of human development. At present, a primary goal of this research is to identify the molecular mechanisms that allow undifferentiated stem cells to differentiate into one of the several hundred different cell types that make up the human body.

Scientists have learned that turning genes on and off is central to this process. But we do not yet fully understand the signals that turn specific genes on and off to influence the differentiation of the stem cell into a specialized cell with a specific function, such as a nerve cell. This knowledge will not only offer the opportunity to learn how to control stem cells from both embryonic and non-embryonic sources, but also provide better understanding of the causes of a number of serious diseases, including those that affect infants and children, which in turn could lead to new and more effective intervention strategies and treatments.

Human stem cells are also being used to speed the development of new drugs. Initially testing thousands of potential drugs on cells in cell culture is typically far more efficient and informative than testing drugs in live animals. *In vitro* systems are useful in predicting *in vivo* responses and provide the benefits of requiring fewer animals, requiring less test material, and enabling higher throughput. New medications can be tested for safety on the specific types of human cells that are affected in disease by deriving these cells from human stem cell lines. Other kinds of cell lines are similarly used in this way. Cancer cell lines, for example, are used to screen potential anti-tumor drugs. The availability of useful stem cell lines would allow drug testing in a wider range of cell types. Potentially, stem cell research will result in a more efficient, effective, safer and faster way of developing drug treatments for a vast array of illnesses, but not until we produce the fundamental discoveries that will pave the way for the widespread use of stem cells in this manner.

Advances in Stem Cell Research

Over the past year, scientists have made remarkable discoveries about the potential of stem cells. For example, NIH-funded scientists have developed a method to coax human embryonic stem cells (hESCs) into becoming cells that resemble lung epithelial cells. The scientists engineered a virus (modified to eliminate its disease-transmitting function) to infect cells with two genes simultaneously, one that drives them into becoming a specialized type of lung cell and another that enables them to resist being killed by a drug (neomycin). Only those cells that express the two genes survived when the scientists treated the culture dish with neomycin. In this way, they were able to generate a pure population of lung-like cells, with no contaminating cells. The surviving cells had the appearance and shape of lung-lining cells called alveolar type 2 cells, which help maximize air exchange, remove fluid from the lungs, serve as a pool of repair cells, and fight airborne diseases. (*Proceedings of the National Academy of Sciences of the USA* 104(11):4449–4454, laboratory of R.A. Wetsel. 2007 March.)

In another experiment, NIH-funded investigators developed a new technique to generate large numbers of pure cardiomyocytes (heart muscle cells) from hESCs. They also formulated a "prosurvival" cocktail (PSC) of factors designed to overcome several known causes of transplanted cell death. The scientists then induced heart attacks in rats and injected the rat hearts with either hESC-derived human cardiomyocytes plus PSC (treatment group) or one of several control preparations. Four weeks later, the scientists identified human cardiomyocytes being supported by rat blood vessels in the treated rat hearts. The treated rat hearts also demonstrated an improved ability to pump blood. The control animals presented no improvement in heart function. This work demonstrates that hESC-derived cardiomyocytes can survive and improve function in damaged rat hearts. Scientists now hope to learn how the human cells improved the rat hearts, and eventually to test this method to treat human heart disease. (*Nature Biotechnology* 25(9):1015–1024, laboratory of CE Murry. 2007 Sept.)

In a significant advance, Japanese scientists and a team of NIH-supported scientists reported that they each succeeded at reprogramming adult human skin cells to behave like hESCs. The Japanese team forced adult skin cells to express the proteins *Oct3/4*, *Sox2*, *Klf4*, and c-Myc, while the NIH-supported team forced adult skin cells to express *OCT4*, *SOX2*, *NANOG*, and *LIN28*. The genes were all chosen for their known importance in maintaining the so-called "stemness" properties of stem cells. In both reports, the adult skin cells are thus reprogrammed into human induced pluripotent stem (iPS) cells that demonstrate important characteristics of pluripotency. The techniques reported by these research teams will enable scientists to generate patient-specific and disease-specific human stem cell lines for laboratory study, and to test potential drugs on human cells in culture. However, these human iPS cells are not yet suitable for use in transplantation medicine. The current techniques use viruses that could generate tumors or other undesirable mutations in cells derived from iPS cells. Scientists are now working to accomplish reprogramming in adult human cells without using potentially dangerous viruses. (*Cell* 131:861–72, laboratory of S. Yamanaka, 2007 Nov 30; *Science* 318:1917–1920, laboratory of J. Thomson, 2007 Dec 21

Researchers from Japan were the first to successfully generate germ cells (the cells that give rise to sperm or eggs) from mouse iPS cells, and their results were verified and extended by another independent laboratory (Rudolf Jaenisch) in the United States. Recent publications from the same Japanese scientists, a team of NIH-supported scientists from University of Wisconsin-Madison, and the Harvard Stem Cell Institute report that they have each succeeded at reprogramming adult human skin cells to become human iPS cells.

There is no doubt that this finding is a remarkable scientific achievement, providing non-embryonic sources of pluripotent cells. Human ESCs and iPS cells are excellent tools to study differentiation, reversal of differentiation, and re-differentiation. In addition, both types of pluripotent cells may be useful for studying the cell biologic changes that accompany human disease. However, from a purely scientific view, it is essential to pursue all types of stem cell research simultaneously, including hESC research, since we cannot predict which type of stem cell will lead to the best possible therapeutic application.

In addition, reprogramming adult human cells would not have been possible without years of prior research studying the properties of hESCs. Two fundamental factors critical to the development of human iPS cells are based upon the knowledge gained from studying hESCs: knowledge of "stemness" genes whose expression or repression is essential to maintain pluripotency; and hESC culture conditions. NIH is proud of the role it has played in supporting this work since 2001 and advancing non-embryonic sources of pluripotent cells.

Scientists must now focus on understanding the mechanism by which retroviral transduction and consequent expression of "stemness" genes induce pluripotency in somatic cells. The consequences of using retroviral vectors to induce pluripotentiality for normal cell functions are unclear, and because the retroviral vectors integrate into the genome of the somatic cell, it can cause the cell to function abnormally. Scientists are now looking for safer methods to reprogram adult cells to a pluripotent state that do not disrupt the genome.

NIH Stem Cell Symposium on Cell-Based Therapies

Two days ago, on May 6, the NIH hosted a symposium entitled "Challenges and Promise of Cell-Based Therapies." Notable stem cell researcher Dr. Stuart Orkin opened the symposium by explaining how 25 years of active research using blood stem cells has led to their successful use in the treatment of blood cancers and other blood disorders. He described the critical characteristics of blood-forming stem cells that have enabled their use in therapies, and how this knowledge will help scientists understand ways to use these and other types of stem cells for treating human diseases. Prominent scientists then discussed how they are developing stem cells as therapies for diseases of the nervous system, heart, muscle and bone, and metabolic disorders. The scientists shared their research results, the technical hurdles they must overcome, and what they ultimately hope to achieve with stem cells. Dr. George Daley of the Harvard Stem Cell Institute gave the final presentation on patient-specific pluripotent stem cells, also known as induced pluripotent stem cells.

Federal Funding of Stem Cell Research

NIH has acted quickly and aggressively to provide support for this research in accordance with the President's 2001 stem cell policy. Since 2001, NIH has invested approximately $3.7 billion on all types of stem cell research. Within this total, NIH has funded: more than $174 million in research studying human embryonic stem cells; more than $1.3 billion on research using human non-embryonic stem cells; more than $628 million on nonhuman embryonic stem cells; and more than $1.5 billion on nonhuman non-embryonic stem cells.

Additionally, in FY 2009, it is projected that NIH will spend approximately $41 million on human embryonic stem cell research and about $203 million on human non-embryonic stem cell research, while also investing approximately $105 million on nonhuman embryonic stem cell research and nearly $306 million on nonhuman non-embryonic stem cell research.

In addition, NIH is conducting activities under the President's July 2007 directive in Executive Order 13435, which directs HHS and NIH to ensure that the human pluripotent stem cell lines on research that it conducts or supports are derived without creating a human embryo for research purposes or destroying, discarding, or subjecting to harm a human embryo or fetus. The order expands the NIH Embryonic Stem Cell registry to include all types of ethically produced human pluripotent stem cells, and renames the registry as the Human Pluripotent Stem Cell Registry. The order invites scientists to work with the NIH, so we can add new ethically derived stem cell lines to the list of those eligible for federal funding.

Further, NIH has encouraged stem cell research through the establishment of an NIH Stem Cell Task Force, a Stem Cell Information Web Site, an Embryonic

Stem Cell Characterization Unit, training courses in the culturing of human embryonic stem cells, support for multidisciplinary teams of stem cell investigators, and a National Stem Cell Bank and Centers of Excellence in Translational Human Stem Cell Research, as well as through extensive investigator initiated research. NIH determined that obtaining access to hESC lines listed on the Human Pluripotent Stem Cell Registry and the lack of trained scientists with the ability to culture hESCs were obstacles to moving this field of research forward. To remove these potential barriers, the National Stem Cell Bank and the providers on the Human Pluripotent Stem Cell Registry together have currently made over 1400 shipments of the hESC cell lines that are eligible for federal funding, as posted on the Human Pluripotent Stem Cell Registry web site. In addition, the NIH-supported hESC training courses have taught several hundred scientists the techniques necessary to culture these cells. We plan to continue to aggressively fund this exciting area of science.

Thank you for the opportunity to present these exciting developments to you. I will be happy to try to answer any questions.

Chapter Sources

The following chapters have been previously published:

Chapter 1 – This is an edited, reformatted and augmented version of a Congressional Research Service publication, Report RS21044, dated March 9, 2009.

Chapter 2 - This is an edited, reformatted and augmented version of a Congressional Research Service publication, Report RL33554, dated March 18, 2009.

Chapter 3 – This is an edited, reformatted and augmented version of a Congressional Research Service publication, Report RL33554, dated March 13, 2009.

Chapter 4 - These remarks were delivered as testimony given on May 8, 2008. Joseph R. Bertino, presented to the House Committee on Energy and Commerce's Subcommittee on Health.

Chapter 5 - These remarks were delivered as testimony given on May, 8, 2008. George Q. Daley, Associate Professor of Biological Chemistry, Medicine, and Pediatrics at Children's Hospital Boston and Harvard Medical School, presented to the House Committee on Energy and Commerce's Subcommittee on Health "Stem Cell Science: The Foundation for Future Cures".

Chapter 6 – These remarks were delivered as testimony given by John K. Fraser, Principal Scientist, Cytori Therapeutics Inc.

Chapter 7 - These remarks were delivered as testimony given on May 8, 2008. John Gearhart for "Stem Cell Science: The Foundation for Future Cures," before the United States House of Representatives Subcommottee on Health of the Committee on Energy and Commerce.

Chapter 8 – These written remarks were delivered as testimony given on May 8, 2008. Weyman Johnson, Individual living with Multiple Sclerosis, Chairman of the Board, National Multiple Sclerosis Society to the Energy and Commerce Committee, Subcommittee on Health, United States House of Representatives, "Stem Cell Science."

Chapter 9 - These remarks were delivered as testimony by Amit N Patel, Director, Cardiovascular Cell Therapies, McGowan Institute of Regenerative Medicine, for "Stem Cell Science: The Foundation for Future Cures" before the Subcommittee on Health of the Committee on Energy and Commerce.

Chapter 10 - This website information has been edited, reformatted and augmented from www.douglastrice.org adult stem cell recipient, presented by Douglas T. Rice, Adult Stem Cell Recipient for the heart, dated May 8, 2008.

Chapter 11 - These remarks were delivered as testimony given on May 8, 2008. Elias A. Zerhouni, Director, National Institutes of Health, United States Department of Health and Human Services, before the Subcommittee on Health Committee on Energy and Commerce United States House of Representatives.

Index

F

G

H

T